# CURRICULUM AND INSTRUCTION IN NURSING

## Concepts and Process

### IMOGENE M. KING

University of South Florida
College of Nursing
*Tampa, Florida*

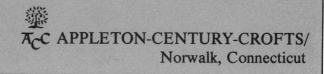
ACC APPLETON-CENTURY-CROFTS/
Norwalk, Connecticut

ISBN    0-8385-1345-X

86  87  88  89  90/  10  9  8  7  6  5  4  3  2  1


Prentice-Hall International (UK) Limited, *London*
Prentice-Hall of Australia Pty. Limited, *Sydney*
Prentice-Hall of Canada Inc., *Toronto*
Prentice-Hall Hispanoamericana, S.A., *Mexico*
Prentice-Hall of India Private Limited, *New Delhi*
Prentice-Hall of Japan, Inc., *Tokyo*
Prentice-Hall of Southeast Asia Pte. Ltd., *Singapore*
Editora Prentice-Hall do Brasil, Ltda., *Rio de Janeiro*
Whitehall Books Limited, *Wellington, New Zealand*


*Library of Congress Cataloging-in-Publication Data*

King, Imogene M.
    Curriculum and instruction in nursing.

    Includes bibliographies and index.
    1. Nursing–Study and teaching.  I. Title.  [DNLM:
1. Curriculum.  2. Education, Nursing.  WY 18 K523c]
RT71.K56  1986      610.73'07'11      85-15737
ISBN  0-8385-1345-X


Editorial production supervision and interior
design: Virginia Huebner
Cover design: 20/20 Services, Inc.
Manufacturiing buyer: John Hall


PRINTED IN THE UNITED STATES OF AMERICA

# Contents

# Preface

This book was written for nurses aspiring to become teachers, for those who are teachers in colleges, schools, and departments of nursing in higher education, and for nurses involved in health teaching. Nurses in staff education positions in health-care systems will find the information useful in designing programs for continuing education and staff development within which courses and modules for selected topics can be developed, presented, and evaluated.

Two schools of thought have prevailed in nursing education since M. Adelaide Nutting implemented the first course to prepare teachers for nursing in 1899 at Teachers College, Columbia University, New York. Nutting, Stewart, McManus, Montag, and others noted that additional educational preparation beyond basic nursing education was essential for nurses who were to be the teachers of students. The second school of thought is that if one is an expert practitioner, one can teach students both formally and informally. The thesis of this book supports the former, because when nurses decided to become teachers in formal educational programs in higher education, they entered a second profession called education. This profession has a body of specific knowledge, skills, and values just as the profession of nursing does.

Nurses who want to become teachers have a need for specific knowledge in nursing and education. They must have, first and foremost, knowledge, skills, and values in professional nursing. They must be able to use the knowledge and skills and promulgate professional values in providing nursing care for individuals, groups, and communities. In addition, they must have some basic knowledge from the profession of education about learning, teaching, and curriculum to facilitate student learning and to develop, implement, and evaluate curricula in nursing programs in community colleges, senior colleges, and universities. This basic knowledge from education is essential to function effectively in the role of a faculty member in higher education.

A systems approach has been used to select and discuss relevant concepts that provide a theoretical basis for curriculum and instruction. These concepts are learning, teaching, curriculum, philosophy, and a conceptual framework. A process for curriculum development is discussed. It is used to demonstrate application of knowledge in building articulated curriculums for associate and baccalaureate degree programs. Ideas for developing a curriculum for nursing as an academic discipline in higher education are presented. Content and process as content are essential ingredients in curriculum and instruction.

This book has been divided into three parts. Part I presents a theoretical basis for curriculum and instruction. Information has been synthesized and relevant concepts selected that are essential knowledge for individuals who develop curricula for tomorrow's world. Three basic concepts—learning, teaching and curriculum—are discussed in Chapter 1. The roles of learner and teacher in educational programs are discussed. These ideas are perceived to be essential knowledge for discussion of a process for developing curricula. Chapter 2 describes one approach to make explicit the philosophical assumptions of a curriculum. Guidelines for use by faculty groups to formulate a philosophy for a curriculum resulted from a national survey of philosophies of nursing education.

The structure for a curriculum has been called a conceptual framework, the organizing elements in a curriculum. The framework flows from the philosophy of nursing education. Functions for the use of a conceptual framework are presented in Chapter 3.

Part II of this book, beginning with Chapter 4, discusses a process for developing a curriculum for nursing in higher education. The process is based on some of the theoretical formulations in Part I about teaching, learning, and curriculum. This process is used to develop a curriculum for a baccalaureate degree program in Chapter 5 and for an associate degree program in Chapter 6. I have used this process effectively in working with faculty groups and as a consultant in curriculum development. One of the problems in nursing education has been articulation from one level of education to another. Chapter 7 offers one approach to facilitate mobility from an associate degree to a baccalaureate degree program. The concepts and processes suggested in the previous chapters are used to demonstrate curriculum revisions in Chapter 8. These concepts and principles can be used in health care agencies for designing continuing education and staff development programs.

A systems approach provided a means of goal identification, outcomes, and feedback relative to measurement of achievement of goals. Nursing as an academic discipline in higher education has come of age. The future has been decided. Part III presents ideas for the structure of a curriculum for nursing as an academic discipline in higher education. Criteria for measuring nursing as a discipline are offered. Chapter 9 suggests a curriculum for the discipline of nursing. Chapter 10 raises questions about research in nursing education.

## ACKNOWLEDGMENTS

An expression of thanks is given to the many authors cited in this volume for their ideas and research in learning, teaching, and curriculum. Thanks is given to my niece, Donna Gwin, for editing the manuscript before it was typed. I am extremely grateful to my sister, Mercedes Fogelson, for her support and for typing the original manuscript. The editors and wonderful people at Prentice-Hall, Inc. have been most helpful.


Tampa, Florida                                    *Imogene M. King chapter*

**1**

# Major Concepts in Curriculum and Instruction

## INTRODUCTION

In a world that proclaims automation, mechanization, high technology, and constant change as a way of life, there is a place for developing, imparting, and evaluating knowledge for decision making in all facets of life. In a world of rapid change, there is also a need for some constants to preserve the values of a culture that maintain the foundation for each society. For many years, American society has promulgated a philosophy that every citizen should have the equality of educational opportunity. When the community college movement of the 1950's began to plan for implementation of this belief, additional social changes were taking place, especially in the area of human rights. Change has become a way of life as we look to the twenty-first century. Change has increased anxiety, and education has been viewed as the way to cope with change and to learn to prepare for a world of work.

The educational system is perceived as a place for planned change in the behavior of citizens. Because education is essential for living and working, the system has been scrutinized, praised, blamed, and studied over the years. Research and development have advanced knowledge and technology, and education is viewed today as a life-long process. Research about learning, teaching, and curriculum has been responsible for some of the changes in the educational system. Part I (Chapter 1, 2 and 3) is a synthesis of studies and reports that propose a systems approach as a theoretical basis for curriculum and instruction.

As a member of several faculty groups and as a curriculum consultant, I know from experience the difficulty encountered in stating a philosophy that guides curriculum development. To some individuals, the first chapter of a book of this type should begin with philosophy. However, it is difficult, if not impossible, to engage in faculty discussions about philosophy without prior knowledge of learning, teaching, curriculum, and roles of learners and teachers. For example, it is difficult to make philosophical pronouncements about the nature of a learner if one has not developed a concept of learning. Since faculty members are teachers, they should have developed their own concepts of teaching. When faculty members' knowledge about learning and teaching is combined with knowledge of curriculum, evaluation, and roles of learner and teacher, a discussion of a statement of philosophy that guides curriculum and instruction is facilitated. For these reasons, the first chapter in this book presents the author's concepts of learning, teaching, curriculum, and role of learner and teacher. Another reason for the organization is that when one is developing a curriculum, the process usually begins with a statement of philosophy, followed by a conceptual framework and program objectives or competencies expected in students upon graduation. This way of organizing the book seemed to present a flow of events in sequence.

Knowledge about learning, teaching, and curriculum is essential for faculty members who are responsible for curriculum development, curriculum revision, and the implementation of instruction in nursing in higher education. These three concepts provide a theoretical basis for curriculum and instruction. The roles of learner and of teacher are viewed as distinct and complementary. Learners and teachers have specific functions to perform in these roles. A few ideas about the role of teacher and role of learner are presented.

## A CONCEPT OF LEARNING

My concept of learning, which is my knowledge about learning, has been developed over many years. I share it with the reader because of a strong belief that if teachers know about learners and learning, curricula would be developed to accommodate learners rather than teachers and the educational system. In developing my concept, a review of theories of learning was an essential first step in gaining knowledge about learning. A review of the studies conducted to test ideas from these theories was a second step. From my analysis of the literature and a synthesis of the findings, a concept has been developed.

The process used for development of each concept includes:

1) a review of the literature, 2) an identification of the characteristics of the concept describing the nature of it, and 3) a definition of the concept. The characteristics and definition are derived from the literature. The knowledge gained from development of a concept is applied in a variety of situations. Concepts and theories are not applied because they are abstractions, but knowledge derived from them is applied.

The following outline is used to develop a concept:

1. Review the literature related to the concept, such as communication theories and studies related to them.

2. Review the nursing literature for studies of the concept; for example, the Daubenmire et al. study (1978).

3. From the above analysis, identify the characteristics of the concept (the nature of it).

4. Write an operational definition of the concept.

Multiple sources are available to read about teaching and learning (Bruner, 1966; Gagne, 1975; Bloom, 1976). Although knowledge about learning, teaching, and curriculum is available to educators, use of this knowledge is not always obvious in the classroom, in the program of studies, and in the total curriculum. In presenting my concept of learning, theories and models are reviewed and learning processes are identified. Characteristics of learning are derived from analysis of the literature. A definition of learning is presented and guidelines for learning are suggested.

## Overview of Theories

Change in human behavior is facilitated by alterations in perceptions. Differential perceptions are responsible for variations in individual and group behavior. Knowledge of perception is central to understanding learning. Learning may occur without directly observable changes in behavior. However, inferences are made that learning has taken place when individuals exhibit changes in concepts, skills, habits, symbols, and values. In designing future studies of learning, one should consider the dependent variable, change in behavior, and experience, the independent variable, as observable even though learning, the intervening variable, is not directly observable.

Research and development have brought about increased emphasis on learning and changes in curricula in elementary, secondary, and higher education. Findings from studies about human learning, remembering, and transfer have indicated movement away from the traditional connectionist and field theories of learning to a systems approach in which learning is the focus of the educational system (Banathy, 1968; Pfeiffer, 1968; Frymier, 1969; Bloom, Hastings, and Madaus, 1971).

Learning theories have been reported and tested for many years. Analysis of the theories and findings of studies indicated that two questions have been consistently and continuously asked. First, how does human learning take place? Second, what factors determine what human beings will learn and how rapidly they will learn it? Psychologists, educators, physiologists and philosophers have been studying, discussing, and writing about these two questions for many years. Computer technology and research in systems theory have provided methods and approaches to deal with multiple variables in concrete situations. Some research findings have been reported in which cognitive mapping is one approach to identify cognitive styles of individuals (Nunney and Hill, 1972). Research findings and techniques related to a concept of mastery learning hold that anyone can learn any task given enough time, guidance, and appropriate learning activities (Bloom, Madaus, and Hastings, 1981). Theories have provided a way of analyzing, discussing, and conducting research about learning. Theories have stimulated scientific thought and summarized knowledge about the way individuals learn. Theories have explained what learning is and why individuals learn what they want to know. Theories have attempted to determine the underlying structure of how we learn about the world in which we live.

For purposes of review, traditional theories of learning have been categorized into two schools of thought: 1) connectionist-behaviorist theories, and 2) cognitive-field theories. Readers who wish to increase knowledge about specific theories should consult sources for details about these theories. Modern theories have adopted a systems approach to learning. Concepts from theories have been identified and compared to show relationships between traditional and modern ideas about learning (Hill, 1977).

The connectionist-behaviorist's view of learning indicated that specific stimuli initially called forth specific responses. Each theory in this school of thought added concepts to the early ideas about learning. Concepts of this school of thought have been identified as:

1. contiguity of stimulus and response

2. reinforcement

3. incentive-motivation factor

4. drive, cue, response, and reward

5. operant conditioning and positive reinforcement

Philosophically, some individuals may disagree with the above concepts, but each one has added to knowledge about learning (Hill, 1977).

The cognitive-field theorists were concerned with knowledge that individuals have about their environment and the way these cognitions determined human behavior. Major concepts of this school of thought were:

1. purposive behaviorism

2. pattern and configuration

3. figure and ground as field

4. life space

5. insight

6. perception (Hill, 1977)

All of these concepts and the studies reported in each school of thought have added to our knowledge of learning. Modern theories and models have extended these traditional ideas (Joyce and Wiel, 1972; Gagne, 1975; Bloom, Madaus, and Hastings, 1981).

Within the past twenty-five years a systems approach has been used in education. Gagne (1975), for example, proposed the use of a modern theory of learning known as information processing theory. He identified eight types of learning, arranged sequentially beginning with a simple form of learning called signal learning. This was followed by stimulus-response learning. Chaining, a sequence of stimulus-response units in skill learning, describes the third type of learning in the sequence. The fourth type, verbal association, is naming a thing or an object. After the naming of a thing, one can begin to discriminate this object from that object. Gagne has described a process whereby an individual builds concepts. The first five types of learning deal with perception of concrete things in the environment, followed by some kind of response and forming a relationship of this new perception with something already experienced. Concept development begins with naming a person, object, or event followed by discriminating one thing from another and then forming a generalization. From concepts, one forms rules about things generally and moves to problem solving.

Gagne's theoretical framework for learning emphasized observable behavior and performance for each type of learning. Each related to a process of input in the learner through stimuli in the environment. In a stimulus situation, transformations occur that lead to output, that is, observable behaviors and performance. In a review of concepts in traditional theories, some relationships exist between the old and the new. For example, sensory perceptions involve stimuli in the environment and are essential for learning to occur. Sensory stimuli and behavioral responses to them are important in understanding how individuals learn.

Reward, reinforcement and motivation are elements that influence learning. An assumption has been made throughout the literature that individuals will be motivated to learn if rewarded for specific responses to specific stimuli. In the process of growth and development, individuals become conscious of goals and come to value them. Identification of one's goals and the means to achieve them influences what one will learn and how quickly. In this sense, achievement of a goal can be assumed to be a reward. This provides reinforcement which increases the motivation to continue to learn because learning helps to achieve goals.

The traditional stimulus-response theory can be compared to the input of information from the external environment in the language of systems. Every system has a goal. Goal, as an element in learning, is derived from the field theorists' concept of purposive behavior. The concepts of figure and ground as field help one understand pattern and configuration and Lewin's concept of life space. Achievement of goals can be related to incentive-motivation factors in Hull and Spence's theoretical formulations, to reward in Dollard and Miller's work, and to reinforcement in Skinner and Thorndike's theories. Pattern and configuration can be elements in the processing of inputs from the environment resulting in outputs in behavior. Gestaltists' "figure and ground as field" theory and Lewin's life space concept are related to individuals' responses as a unified whole. These ideas make assumptions about the way individuals respond as a unified whole to the field, which indicates that a concept of perception is essential for learning. The relationship between the concepts of traditional theories and modern theories provides a basis for understanding how individuals learn. This knowledge is useful in curriculum and instruction.

## A Systems Approach

Information processing models were designed as part of research and development of complex man-machine systems (Ashby, 1966; Churchman, 1968; Wiener, 1967). Information processing models are rooted in logic, communications, psychology, and neurophysiology. One of the original models is shown in Figure 1.1. This simple model indicates that information from the environment was taken in through the senses and trans-

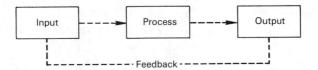

**Figure 1.1**
Information Processing Model

mitted by way of the nervous system to the brain where a percept was formed and perception resulted. This information is categorized as concepts and stored in the memory for recall at a later time when the situation demands the information. Factors that influence perception are shown in Figure 1.2. The output or behavioral manifestations provide feedback as input into the system. Feedback implies that a system is self-regulating. Behavior can be observed and measured directly when educators have identified elements that are required for performance of specific behaviors.

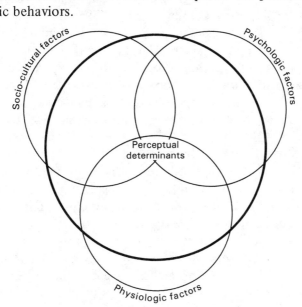

**Figure 1.2**
Factors that Influence Perception (From: I.M. King, *Towards a Theory for Nursing.* New York: John Wiley, 1971, p. 96.)

The systems approach has been used to plan, implement, and evaluate systems as a whole. Every system has a purpose or goal. Purpose determines the processes which are the functions of the system. One function of the educational system is to provide opportunities for learning. To accomplish this function, it is necessary to know about processes involved in learning.

### Learning Processes

The performance of specific behaviors is identified in clearly stated objectives. Taxonomies of educational objectives have been formulated for the cognitive, affective, and psychomotor domains of learning. An experience taxonomy has been published as the most recent categorization about learning. (Steinaker and Bell, 1979). The processes involved in these domains of learning have been identified in the taxonomies (Bloom et al., 1956; Krathwohl, Bloom, and Masia, 1964; Simpson, 1966; Steinaker and Bell, 1979) and are shown in Table 1.1. These processes classify the way that individuals gain knowledge, skills, and values. The experiential taxonomy emphasizes active participation through multiple experiences and is an approach to show the interrelationships of the domains of learning in experience. An observation is made that perception is a common concept in all of these classification systems.

**Cognitive Domain.** In formal educational programs dealing with knowledge, emphasis has been given to the cognitive domain. In using an information processing model for learning, a dual purpose is achieved. Students acquire useful information called content and also develop process skills, one of which is thinking. Learners are active processors of information rather than passive recipients of the teacher's knowledge. Teaching strategies focus on the learners' involvement in gathering and analyzing data from a variety of sources to interpret and form generalizations and abstractions about the world around them. The goal in this approach is to attain information. The diagram in Figure 1.3 shows the processes involved in learning to think. The cognitive processes are observation, measurement, and inference.

**Table 1.1.**

Processes in the Four Domains of Knowledge

## DOMAINS OF KNOWLEDGE

| COGNITIVE[a] | AFFECTIVE[b] | PSYCHOMOTOR[c] | EXPERIENCE[d] |
|---|---|---|---|
| Knowing | Perceiving | Perception | Exposure |
| Comprehending | Responding | Set | Participating |
| Applying | Valuing | Guided response | Indentification |
| Analyzing | Organizing | Mechanism | Internalization |
| Synthesizing | Characterization | Complex overt response | Dissemination |
| Evaluating | | | |

[a]Bloom, et al., *Taxonomy of Educational Objectives: Cognitive Domain*. New York: David McKay, 1956.

[b]Krathwohl, et al., *Taxonomy of Educational Objectives: Affective Domain*. New York: David McKay, 1964.

[c]Simpson, E.J., *The Classification of Educational Objectives: Psychomotor Domain*. Urbana, Ill.: University of Illinois Press, 1966.

[d]Steinaker, N.W., and Bell, M.R., *The Experiential Taxonomy: A New Approach to Teaching and Learning*. New York: Academic Press, 1979.

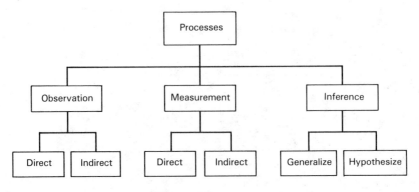

**Figure   1.3**
Cognitive Processes

**Observation.**   One way of knowing about our world is observation, which is a process for gathering empirical facts through sensory experiences in our environment. All science begins with observation of events in the environment. Two types of observation, direct and indirect, have been identified. Direct observation is gathering information about objects, persons, and events and is called raw sensory data. Indirect observation is gathering information about objects, persons, and events through sources other than direct sensory experiences such as books, newspapers, and written records. To assure accuracy in one's observations, planned experiences in observing and quantifying observations can help individuals acquire observation skills and gather accurate information about the world. Observation has been used to gather scientific information. Two methods, participant and nonparticipant observations, have been employed to gather data. Consult sources for further information about observation. (Bruyn, 1966; Webb et al., 1966; Bogdan and Taylor, 1975).

**Measurement.**   Measurement is another way to gather information directly and indirectly. Measurement has a connotation of being more precise and objective than observations, but this is not necessarily a valid assumption. The term implies that instruments are used to gather objective information in a systematic way. An example of direct measurement would be to determine the number of red and white blood cells from an individual's blood sample. An example of an indirect measure is taking a person's blood pressure.

**Inference.** From information gathered through observations and measurement, inferences are made about events in the environment. Inferences are interpretations made by individuals from a few observations or measurements or from many observations and measurements. A type of inference made by individuals generally and by researchers specifically is hypothesizing. If a teacher expects learners to acquire critical thinking skills, experiences must be planned for learners to practice making inferences to recognize the validity of the inferences and to verify the accuracy of the inferences. When individuals are learning the processes of observation, measurement, and inference, content is also learned. The diagram in Figure 1.4 indicates that content and process are essential to achieve goals.

Concrete information gathered in the environment has been called facts. Multiple facts about similar phenomena provide information whereby individuals begin to classify bits of information into categories or concepts. Concepts are developed from multiple experiences with concrete things. From concepts, individuals form generalizations about the world. Learning content is brought about by gathering facts, developing abstractions

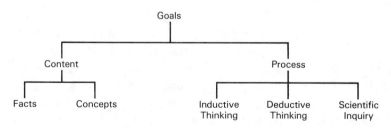

**Figure 1.4**
Cognitive Domain—Content and Process

or concepts from the facts, and drawing conclusions by making some generalizations about the facts. This is called knowledge.

The teacher provides information that the learners can process into concepts and generalizations that have meaning for them. Acquisition of knowledge requires intellectual skills. These skills are developed through the use of inductive and deductive reasoning and logical thinking. Inductive reasoning is a mental process whereby conclusions to particular ideas are drawn from general laws or principles. As students learn a process of thinking, they are also gaining knowledge, which is content. Process and content are interrelated and complementary in a systems approach to learning.

Thinking involves sensations that differ in quality, intensity, and duration based on the disposition of the learner and the environment in which learning takes place. Perception gives meaning to sensory experiences through the process of interpreting sensations. Perceptual experiences build concepts. A concept is an abstract representation of persons, objects, and things in the world. Concepts are the ideas that are stored in one's memory for recall at a later time. There are two classifications of ideas: 1) universal ideas represent common characteristics of a thing, a person, or an object, such as, a chair, a human being, the weather; 2) particular ideas represent a specific object, person, or thing, such as, this patio chair, John and Mary, my red pencil. Conceptualizing one's world results in knowledge. Problem solving is a systematic method of gathering, analyzing, and interpreting information. This technique is one approach in learning a process of inquiry. Content results in facts, concepts, and generalizations.

Processes involved in the affective domain overlap with those in the cognitive domain. There are complex relationships between the cognitive and affective domains. The individuals who developed the taxonomies believed that the cognitive and affective domains of learning are interrelated. The relationship between the taxonomy categories of the cognitive and affective domains is described in the initial work of these groups (Krathwohl, Bloom, and Masia, 1964). This separation was done to place emphasis on identification of affective objectives and to evaluate learning that deals with interests, appreciations, and values. If teachers believe that intended outcomes in the affective domain are an essential component in learning, then affective objectives must be formulated and evaluated. Continued research is needed to understand the nature of each domain and the relationship of one to the other.

**Affective Domain.** The processes involved in affective learning overlap with some of those involved in cognitive learning because human beings perceive objects, persons, and events in their environment selectively. So, too, in learning experiences planned in formal educational programs, individuals control the stimuli in the environment. This process is known as selective perception. A second process is response to stimuli. In the affective domain, this response includes accepting responsibility for events in the world and gaining satisfaction in one's responses. Valuing is a third process in which individuals accept some events and behaviors as having worth and organize them into a system of values. A final category in the affective domain is called characterization. At this point in the learning process, individual behaviors can be observed and identified as characterizing an individual's values and a specific philosophy of life. The relationships between the cognitive objectives may become the means to achieve affective goals, and vice versa. (Krathwohl, Bloom, and Masia, 1964). These two domains are also related to the psychomotor domain of learning, because skills require knowledge and feeling for action. These domains have been separated to place emphasis on specific components of the learning process in human beings.

**Psychomotor Domain.** This domain of learning emphasizes motor activity. Perception is essential in performing a motor act. Perception is defined as a process of organizing, interpreting and transforming information from sense data and memory to give meaning to one's experience, represent one's image of reality, and influence one's behavior (King, 1981, pp. 20, 24). In the act of perceiving, one must be aware of stimuli, then attend to

them and select or control the input of stimuli. In the performance of a task, cues in the situation, knowledge, and past experiences are selected as guides to action. A mental process is
required to relate perception to action in performing a motor
act. Readiness for an experience with some kind of action has
been called "set." Mental set deals with knowledge of steps in a
motor activity; physical set focuses attention on the body and
position; emotional set involves an attitude or desire to perform
the motor act.

A third process in the psychomotor domain is guided response in the development of a skill. The learner is under the
guidance of a teacher. One approach, imitation, is performing
an act in the same way the teacher demonstrates it. Another
way is by trial and error, whereby multiple responses are tried
until one selects the response that meets performance requirements.

Mechanism is a fourth category in the psychomotor domain of learning. This category indicates that the learner has
acquired confidence and skill in performance of a motor act.
The learned response becomes habitual.

The fifth category in the performance of motor activities
is called a complex overt response. The learner is able to perform
complex movement patterns efficiently and effectively. Uncertainty in performance is resolved at this state and individuals
perform complex motor skills automatically.

The designers of the taxonomies of educational objectives
have indicated they are a classification of behaviors which represent "intended outcomes of the educational process" (Bloom,
et al., 1956). These categories have been used here as a classification of learning processes rather than outcomes. The outcomes are those statements of specific objectives to be achieved
by learners from knowledge of these processes.

Before stating specific objectives to be attained by learners,
teachers use information available to assess learning styles and
to assess prerequisite knowledge of learners to plan for meeting individual differences. For many years, educators have
viewed personality, emotions, and motivation of learners as
essential factors in learning. Over the past ten years, research

findings have provided information about the assessment of learning styles of individuals. Learning styles have been described as 1) visual or reading; 2) aural or listening; and 3) physical or doing things. No two individuals learn the same things in the same way at the same rate of speed. Some individuals learn more easily through reading or listening or doing things. Some persons work best under pressure of deadlines and tests. Others must adopt a more leisurely pace. Some individuals learn more easily by being challenged by those with greater knowledge or by helping those with less knowledge.

**Cognitive Mapping.** Joseph Hill identified a way to test learners to discover their cognitive style (1967). He and his colleagues have designed a battery of tests to determine cognitive mapping. Four components are identified by the tests.

1. Theoretical symbolic orientation is identified through verbal aptitude tests, IQ tests, reading, and mathematics tests.

2. Qualitative symbolic orientation is identified through auditory, olefactory, taste, touch, visual, proprioceptive, code-empathetic, code-ethic, code-histrionic, code-kinesics, code-proxemics, code-synnoetics, and code-transactional means.

3. Cultural determinants are identified through information about family, individuals, and associates.

4. Modalities of inference and forms of inference the individual uses in the process of deriving meaning have been delineated.

   a. categorical thinking uses norms.

   b. D-difference deals with comparison of selected measurements.

   c. R-relationship deals with relation between one or more measurements.

          d. L-appraisal type of inference considers with equal
            weight the hypotheses of above in arriving at a con-
            clusion (Nunney and Hill, 1972, pp. 10–15).

With these kinds of tests available to determine cognitive mapping
for individual learners, one questions why this approach has not
been adopted more widely in educational programs.

    Cognitive mapping is one approach to use to match the
cognitive style of learning with the various teaching strategies to
facilitate the learner's success in educational endeavors. The
task of the teacher is to match his or her mode of presentation
of information to the cognitive style of the learner to develop a
"personalized educational program" for learners. Such a program promotes learner success because it enhances the learner's
"personal educational prescription" (Nunney and Hill, 1972,
p. 11). Learning processes described here lead to learning outcomes.

### Learning Outcomes

    When processes are focused on learners rather than teachers,
specific concepts, skills and values are identified as essential for
learners. A traditional set of expectations by teachers at all
levels of education has shown that outcomes were based on the
"normal curve": about one-third of the students would achieve
the outcomes expected; one-third would be average; one-third
of the students would just pass; and some would fail. According
to Bloom and colleagues (1971), this set of expectations is costly,
destructive, and wasteful; use of the normal curve in grading
students' achievement today is no longer valid and should be
abolished. Bloom and colleagues (1971) found that more than
90% of students can master any subject a teacher can teach
given specific objectives, appropriate learning materials, and
time.

### Mastery Learning

Bloom and colleagues (1971) identified five variables which influence an approach to building a curriculum for mastery learning.

First, students are individuals and have aptitudes for particular kinds of learning. In the past, aptitude tests were viewed as good predictors of achievement. Carroll, however, put forth a contrasting view when he stated, "Aptitude is the amount of time required by the learner to attain mastery of a learning task" (Carroll, 1963). Bloom and colleagues (1971) extended Carroll's ideas and noted "that aptitudes are predictive of rate of learning rather than level of complexity of learning." They indicated that given "sufficient time and appropriate types of help, 95% of the students can learn a subject with a high degree of mastery" (p. 46).

Second, Bloom and colleagues noted quality of instruction as another variable that influences what students will learn. Carroll (1963) defined quality of instruction as related to the presentation of the tasks to be learned. Since each learner is an individual, the teacher has a responsibility to sequence the tasks to be learned in a way that they are optimum for any learner. In this sense, quality of instruction is not only the instructional materials, the teacher, or the curriculum but the specificity with which the teacher presents and explains clearly the expectations for the learner, and the learner relates to the tasks to be learned (p. 47).

Third, the ability to understand instruction deals with the student-teacher interactions with the instructional materials and the procedures to follow to learn the task. Materials include verbal information, textbooks, workbooks, formative evaluation procedures and tutorial help (pp. 48-49).

Fourth, the learner's perseverance influences mastery and refers to the time the learner is willing to spend in learning the tasks identified. The quality of learning is related to attitudes, interests, and goals of learners. When resources for learning are planned by teachers to reduce learning time, this planning tends to facilitate achievement of tasks to be learned (p. 50).

Fifth, time allowed for learning has been traditionally planned in most school systems to provide group instruction for definite periods of time in which all learners are expected to learn the tasks. Carroll (1963) noted that the time spent on learning is the key to mastery. He believed that the student, given enough time to learn, could achieve mastery. This kind of change in school systems involves organization as well as instruction. In addition, it involves continuing education for teachers to understand this approach to their role and functions (p. 51).

Implementation of mastery learning in a curriculum requires two types of evaluation. First, formative evaluation is an integral part of planning curricula for mastery learning. This evaluation involves specific objectives, content of instruction, and learning tasks that teachers and students are expected to do to achieve the tasks. Formative evaluation procedures are an integral part of guiding learners through learning activities. Formative evaluation must be clearly defined as the appraisal of learners as part of the teacher-learning process and is not used for grading purposes, but for guiding learners to achieve the tasks.

Summative evaluation identifies procedures that are used to measure outcomes of instruction. Measurement of learning outcomes tells teachers and students that the instruction has been effective. Summative evaluation is appraisal of the achievement or performance of students at the completion of a module or of a course and is used for grading.

Specific concepts have been identified for teachers who design and implement programs for mastery learning. Relating individual differences to the teaching-learning process is a basic problem in developing strategies for mastery learning. Several strategies have been identified, such as, tutorial, self-pacing, nongraded programs, and diagnostic procedures and alternative instructional methods and materials. These approaches assist in bringing a large part of the group to a predetermined standard of achievement.

One begins with identifying what is expected of the learner; that is, one defines mastery and established criteria for mastery learning in a specific module or course. Information is collected to determine if the learners have attained mastery. Specific objectives must be identified and content related to objectives to inform both the teacher and the student what is expected for mastery learning. Evaluation measures are designed to evaluate outcomes of instruction. Teachers must distinguish between learning processes and evaluation processes. The critical elements are identified and serve as the performance criteria, so each student is judged on individual performances against known criteria rather than by his or her rank in a group. This approach recognizes differences among individual learners.

A review of Bloom and colleagues approach to learning for mastery indicated they had discovered a way to emphasize success in learning. Content and learning opportunities are related to behavioral outcomes expected in learners. Processes are focused on learners rather than on teachers. Specific concepts and techniques are essential to teach for mastery.

Gagne (1975) identified five categories of learning outcomes. The end results of achieving behavioral objectives are: 1) verbal information; 2) intellectual skill; 3) cognitive strategy, 4) attitude; and 5) motor skill (p. 68). He noted that one directly observes the performance of learners but must make inferences about learning based on that performance. Human performance is shown in behavioral objectives described by action verbs such as demonstrate, identify, classify, choose, state, list, specify, and differentiate. These elements in learning are essential in planning for instruction.

Generally, the outcomes of learning result in knowing one's strengths and focusing attention on areas to be improved. The application of knowledge will verify its usefulness and reinforce and refine what one already knows. Conceptual knowledge is retained and can be recalled in new situations. In order to facilitate the learning processes to attain learning outcomes, a climate for learning is established.

## Climate for Learning

An atmosphere of incentive and opportunity is conducive to learning. A climate that is free from threat without being free from challenge is essential for learning. When learners have a feeling of acceptance and belonging, they tend to set goals. Learners need teachers who will help them accept success, which is one kind of positive reinforcement that tends to motivate learners to continue to learn. Learners have a need for recognition by peers and teachers. A climate that is flexible will help meet individual differences in learners.

From this review of major concepts from traditional theories of learning, new relationships have been suggested in a presentation of a modern information processing view of learning. In addition, several processes of learning concepts, skills, and values have been suggested. This analysis of views about learning has helped to identify some of the characteristics of learning.

## Characteristics of Learning

Characteristics describe the nature of learning. The following characteristics have been derived from the many individuals who have studied learning and from learning theories and models:

1. *Self activity* is a characteristic that indicates the learner's involvement in the process. No one can learn for another person. The active participation of the learner indicates that learning is individualized. Involvement in multiple activities that meet a learner's purposes will facilitate achievement of goals. Learning is somewhat selective because an individual will learn that which will help him or her achieve goals. Motivation may be influenced by teachers who assist learners to identify purposes.

2. *Perception*, as an integral component in the learning process, is a characteristic of learning. Individuals re-

ceive multiple stimuli from their environment which provide perceptual experiences from which concepts are developed. Learning requires sensory experiences in the act of perceiving one's world. Without perceptual experiences, learning would be limited. Perceiving is a process that has been identified in each of the domains of learning.

3. *Communication* is a characteristic of learning and is the information component of human interactions. Learning requires information, which is provided through verbal or nonverbal messages.

4. *Transaction* is a characteristic of learning and is the valuational component of human interactions. When a person values something, that individual makes transactions with other persons to achieve goals.

5. *Goal orientation* signifies that one will learn that which has purpose for the individual and helps achieve goals. Learning is individual because it is goal directed. Each learner tends to learn that which helps him or her achieve immediate and long range goals. Learners bring personal interests, needs, and past experiences to learning situations. The learning climate may enhance or detract from achievement of goals.

6. *Dynamic* is a characteristic that describes the learning process as ongoing change as each new experience increases information input.

7. *Feedback* describes learning as a self-regulating process because the outcome of learning may serve as input for future learning. Learning requires feedback in the processing of information which verifies one's perceptions. Reinforcement through feedback provides verification for learners and gives satisfaction in achievement of goals.

8. *Personal* is a term that characterizes learning, because each learner exhibits different wants, needs, and goals.

9. *Conceptual* describes a kind of cognitive learning. Learning concepts provides a storehouse of information for retention and recall for transfer to a new situation at a later time.

10. *Affective* describes feelings involved in learning. Learning is influenced by feelings and emotions.

11. *Psychomotor* describes motor activity. Motor acts involve skill in performance and reduce uncertainty.

12. *Thinking* is an essential component in learning. Learning involves deductive and inductive reasoning, analysis, interpretation, synthesis, and judgments.

From these characteristics, the following definition of learning has been formulated.


## Definition of Learning

Learning is a process of sensory perception, conceptualization, and critical thinking involving multiple experiences in which changes in concepts, skills, symbols, habits, and values can be evaluated in observable behaviors and inferred from behavioral manifestations.

Each learner develops, grows, and learns as a whole person. Each learner has a unique background of experiences; therefore, teachers must recognize and plan for individual differences in learning. Each individual learns at his or her own pace. Each individual brings to a learning situation his or her own self-concept, feeling of personal worth, and ways of protecting and maintaining self-respect. Above all, each person brings to a learning situation his or her own purposes, goals, and motives, which are complex and varied. Each individual has a different readiness for learning and a different learning style.

## Guidelines for Learning About Learning

The following propositions about learning will serve a useful purpose for faculty groups that develop curricula and plan instruction.

1. Learning is facilitated through planned educational experiences to achieve specific objectives.

2. Learning is facilitated when learners are active and individual learning styles are considered.

3. Learning is efficient and effective when there is feedback, reinforcement, and satisfaction.

4. Learning is influenced by a climate that provides freedom for learning.

5. Learning is influenced by a learner's interests, goals, and attitudes.

6. Learning to develop concepts provides a way to retain knowledge and to transfer knowledge from one situation to another.

A relationship between learning and teaching has been discussed by many individuals. The diagram that shows the interaction is:

$$\text{Teaching} \langle ---- \rangle \text{Learning}$$

This connotes a reciprocal relationship between teaching and learning and indicates the influence of one on the other. Complexities in teaching and learning arise from the educational environment of a community college or a university in which external factors of finance, laws, or societal pressures influence curricula and the teaching-learning process. Internal factors related to the organizational structure of the educational system, such as faculty, administrators, and committees, exert power in the decision-making process.

Faculty members in higher education who have knowledge about learners, the learning process, and the subject to be taught, develop course objectives, learning experiences, and evaluations of learners' achievements based on that knowledge. A concept of teaching is presented to show relationships between teaching and learning.

## A CONCEPT OF TEACHING

A system for teaching deals with the processes embodied in human learning. A systems approach provides for information input, which is a process that exposes students to a body of knowledge, and the meaning, significance, and usefulness of information.

In the past and in some schools today, teaching has been conceived as an act of telling students what they need to know to pass courses and to be promoted to the next level in the educational system. Teaching has been planned for the average student and has assumed a normal distribution in student populations. These two assumptions about teaching are no longer valid because of knowledge about how people learn and about individual learning styles and learning outcomes.

Two terms, *teaching* and *instruction*, are used interchangeably in some writings, and in others they are specifically defined. Some authors discuss theories of instruction and some discuss models of teaching. A dictionary definition of teaching states it is a process of imparting knowledge and instruction directing people's learning by teaching them. Teaching and instruction are used synonomously throughout this book.

Theories of instruction, models of teaching, teaching processes, a climate for teaching, and teaching outcomes are analyzed to develop a concept of teaching. Characteristics of teaching are derived from analysis of the literature. A definition of teaching is presented and guidelines for teaching are suggested.

## Theories and Models of Instruction

Several theories of instruction have been selected for review. Woodruff (1961) suggested that a construct of teaching contained three essential elements: 1) an objective that produces a specific outcome; 2) a learning experience planned for students to achieve the specific outcome stated in the objective; and 3) receptivity to the learning experience planned to attain the objective (p. 30). He noted that a teacher can merely express his or her own concept by talking about it because the meaning of something is unique to each individual and cannot be transmitted per se. It can be communicated as information to another person by a set of symbols, such as words. He stated that teaching is a "process of guiding students through a learning process which is psychologically correct for the thing to be learned" (p. 116). For example, teaching for concept development is different from teaching for skill development. Learning a concept requires seeing or perceiving a referent in one's concrete environment, thinking about it, trying it out, and noting its usefulness. Learning a skill requires practice. Woodruff's construct of teaching is clear, specific, and useful. He has provided some of the basic ideas, which subsequent writers have expanded and extended.

Maccia (1967) proposed a descriptive theory of instruction. She defined formal instruction as "the interaction of teaching and learning within the school" (p. 132). She presented several concepts as important in formal instruction within the school. She described group dynamics in the classroom between learner and teacher as one way to advance knowledge of interpersonal relations. She believed that these relationships implied influence and that decisions should be made about what kind of influence is useful in a teaching-learning situation. Concepts of reward, punishment, legitimacy, expertise, and affect were identified.

A second dimension of Maccia's theory was the discipline approach to curriculum (p. 135). She suggested several meanings for the term discipline. For example, she indicated that discipline could be defined as controlling through authority or punishment. She also believed that discipline is an organized body of knowledge or rules of conduct that could be utilized in her ideas about "rule governed behavior." Instruction to Maccia meant bringing about change in someone by rules regulating and controlling the process.

Maccia emphasized two major ideas in a theory of formal instruction: 1) problem solving about living; and 2) knowledge of the structure of the subject (p. 137). She indicated that teachers must have knowledge of the content they teach and experience in problem solving.

Instruction is one approach to assist individuals to grow, learn, and change. Bruner (1966) noted that a theory of instruction should be concerned with organizing the environment to provide for optimum learning. He believed that a theory of instruction should be congruent with one's theory of intellectual development. Before explicating a theory, he discussed the way in which individuals process information. Initially, young persons know their world by actions, that is, how to do something. Doing is followed by the experiences the individual encounters and the way his or her perceptions, which represent images of things in the environment, categorize these experiences into concepts and generalizations. A third way is through the use of language, which is referred to as symbolic operations. In the process of intellectual growth, individuals organize their thoughts through reflection and state propositions to show relationships about what is known. Bruner stated that the "theory of instruction, in short, is concerned with how what one wishes to teach can best be learned, with improving rather than describing learning" (p. 40).

Bruner's theory of instruction had four components: 1) individuals have a predisposition for learning; 2) knowledge should be structured to be easier to learn; 3) sequencing knowledge provides an effective way to learn; and 4) the nature and pacing of rewards are important (pp. 40–42). Bruner noted that a theory of instruction that is normative and prescriptive improves teaching, facilitates learning, and must be concerned with the learning environment. Teachers must understand the process of knowing because learning experiences are planned on the basis of how one learns a particular behavior.

## Models for Teaching

Several conceptual models for teaching focused on teacher and learner verbal interactions in the classroom (Bellack, 1963; Flanders, 1967). The Flanders system of interaction analysis has been used in describing and analyzing verbal interactions between teacher and students. This system recognized a concept of influence and related it to the direct and indirect influence of the verbal interactions of the teacher in the classroom. A ten category system was identified as follows: 1) accepting student feelings; 2) giving praise; 3) accepting, clarifying, or making use of students' ideas; 4) asking questions; 5) lecturing and giving facts or opinions; 6) giving directions; 7) giving criticism; 8) student responses; 9) student initiation; and 10) confusion or silence. Seven of the ten categories are teacher-directed verbal interactions. Direct influence of teacher-directed learning activities lessens the freedom of the students to interact with the teacher. Indirect influence would have the opposite effect and give students the freedom to respond.

Bellak and associates conducted a descriptive study of the linguistic behavior of teachers and students in secondary schools in a large metropolitan city (1963). Empirical data was classified into pedagogical moves from which patterns were designated as teaching cycles. The structuring and soliciting pedagogical moves were called initiating maneuvers and formed one teaching cycle. The responding and reacting pedagogical moves were called reflexive maneuvers and comprised a second type of teaching cycle. The pattern of communication in the classroom was teacher-to-students and dealt with teacher solicitation and student response. The importance of using questions as a teacing strategy in the classroom was identified in the data. The categories in Bellak's study described the tripartite relationship among teacher, student, and content and served as a theoretical framework for continued testing of ideas related to teaching.

Several models of teaching have been proposed that relate

to cognition. Hickey and Newton's study (1967) of the logical structure of teaching within the field of programmed learning has some relevance for cognitive theory and for a theoretical framework for organizing content to be taught into basic elements and complex concepts. They proposed a logic tree model and emphasized the fact that some content areas can be organized in this manner better than others. This way of organizing content requires the learner to proceed with basic elements and to use a process of analysis while advancing to high-order levels ending with knowing the process of synthesis in order to arrive at knowledge of complex concepts (p. 76–84).

Suchman (1967) developed a theoretical model to help learners acquire the process of scientific inquiry. He noted that learners filter what they take in from the environment and compare it with previous experiences. He suggested that teachers encourage inquiry by creating a climate in which students have the freedom to ask questions and express and test ideas. Teachers should give learners some direction or purpose for their experiences. This mode of inquiry places emphasis on learner initiation of ideas rather than teacher-initiated, -directed, and -controlled learning experiences. Suchman indicated that the inquiry process leads to continuous learning for the future. This model uses both the inductive and deductive approaches to teaching. The teacher identifies goals, selects a program, presents it, formulates hypotheses, and gathers data, analyzes findings, and brings closure on the process. To determine if learners have achieved goals, process and content are evaluated by teacher.

Models of teaching were described clearly by Joyce and Weil (1972). One kind of model explained concept attainment; another described social inquiry; another was the group model distinguishing training groups from other learning groups. They noted that

> learning is viewed as a transaction between the learner and the environment in which neither can be regarded as fixed. . . . Teaching is not just information dissemination and retrieval, it is a human relations problem in which teacher and learner explore and diagnose the needs for and resistances to learning and change (p. 80).

Models designed to aid in information processing were identified. Such models emphasized intellectual abilities and dealt with the cognitive domain. The developmental studies by Piaget described intellectual processes. The Taba model emphasized the process of problem solving from an inductive approach. Two learning theorists' models were Ausubel's theory of meaningful verbal learning and Bruner's ideas about how individuals learn concepts. The summary of ideas about concept attainment indicated that we develop concepts to classify objects, persons, and events, which reduces the necessity for constant learning of the same things each time they are experienced. The models of teaching identified and discussed by Joyce and Weil are helpful for teachers as they plan, implement, and evaluate curriculum and instruction.

Carroll's model (1963) for mastery learning showed that the teacher is the major influence in manipulating external variables, such as resources, environment, and learning opportunities. His thesis was that aptitude is the amount of time required to achieve mastery of the specific learning tasks identified by teachers. This assumption implied that given enough time, guidance, and adequate teaching materials and environment, all learners can achieve mastery. So, the concepts in this model of teaching for mastery learning are: 1) aptitude, which is in contrast to the old way of viewing aptitude; 2) learning opportunities, which are planned to achieve specific goals, are available for all learners, and are guided by teachers through feedback and corrective action during the learning process; 3) ability to understand instruction, which relates to differences in students, some of whom learn well verbally and others who learn physically; 4) perseverance, which is related to a student's willingness to spend time learning the tasks to achieve goals and which implies that, given time, almost all students can master the learning tasks; 5) quality of instruction, which relates to selecting the learning opportunities, selecting appropriate learning materials, sequencing the learning tasks, and providing formative evaluation in the process of learning the tasks. Carroll maintained that this model focused on learners' needs and styles and provided the environment and learning resources for all students to be able to achieve a high level of mastery. The main elements in methods of instruction for mastery learning are to present materials that will help the majority of students attain mastery and to relate teaching processes to individual differences in students (pp. 723–733).

Bloom and colleagues (1971) extended Carroll's ideas about mastery learning. Bloom (1976) later proposed a theory of school learning and conducted studies to determine the variables that influence learning in school. One of the conclusions was that "what any person in the world can learn, almost all persons can learn if provided with appropriate prior and current conditions of learning" (p. 7).

The variables in Bloom's theory were: 1) cognitive entry behaviors; 2) affective entry behaviors; and 3) quality of instruction (p. 161). Entry behaviors imply some form of diagnostic assessment to determine if learners have the prerequisite knowledge to enter into a new learning task. Formative evaluation is a necessary element in implementing a mastery learning curriculum. Studies have been reviewed and conducted by Bloom indicating that learners who do not have the essential prerequisite cognitive behaviors will take more time and guidance to achieve mastery in the next learning task. Prerequisite knowledge, a key variable in accounting for learning of students, must be considered in curriculum development and instruction if students are to be given an opportunity to learn effectively in schools.

Affective entry behaviors are more difficult to assess because they deal with the age of the learner and previous learning experiences. Success and failure in learning in the past influences affective behaviors. Bloom cited studies that indicated that positive affective entry behaviors accounted for 25 percent higher learning achievement than negative behaviors. Affective and cognitive entry behaviors are related. He noted that "up to two-thirds of the variance on achievement measures can be accounted for by the combined effects of affective and cognitive entry behaviors."

The third variable, quality of instruction, identified four major elements for which teachers should be responsible. First, cues from students and the environment require teacher sensitivity and response to the students. Second, active participation of the learner is essential, and the teacher has a responsibility to help learners participate. Third, reinforcement at stages in the learning process is essential. This reinforcement may come from the teacher, the environment, and the internal resources of the students. Fourth, feedback from the teacher may also be considered an external type of reinforcement. It is a way of providing information to learners about their achievement in the process of learning a task. At the time of feedback, teachers may introduce some corrective action in students' learning.

Bloom concluded that the goal of schools is "equality of learning outcomes." His ideas suggested a new philosophy of education. In summary, studies that tested hypotheses generated by Bloom's theory have given the educational system at every level of the educational ladder an approach that could revolutionize teaching and learning in the United States. Findings from research have indicated that all individuals can learn when they are given enough time, instructional materials they can understand, and guidance from teachers. The emphasis is on the learner and learning, with great responsibility on the teacher for planning, implementing, and evaluating learning and achievement. Several processes are involved in teaching.

### Teaching Processes

Teaching is a complex process that facilitates learning. Process is defined as a dynamic function of systems and provides for exchanges of matter and energy through information (King, 1981, p. 69). Teaching is described as a set of processes that can be categorized into three major elements, shown in Figure 1.5.

**Planning.** The teacher is responsible for planning activities named in Figure 1.6. Planning begins with assessing learning needs and diagnosing learning styles. Another element in planning is the establishment of goals from which specific objectives are stated in terms of behaviors expected in students. Clearly

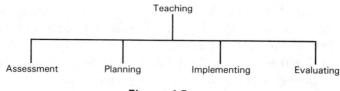

Figure  1.5
Teaching Processes

stated behavioral objectives provide guides for selection of learning activities for students to practice the behaviors expected in achievement of the objectives. For example, if a behavior is in the cognitive domain, experiences would be selected for students to learn facts, concepts, and generalizations.

**Objectives.** Many years ago, Tyler (1949) proposed an approach for formulating clear and concise objectives. His ideas are in use today and have been extended by colleagues in the development of taxonomies of educational objectives. A systematic approach to teaching and learning was influenced by the work of Bloom et al. (1956), Krathwohl et al., (1964), and Simpson (1966) in designing a taxonomy of educational objectives in the cognitive, affective, and psychomotor domains of learning. The taxonomies not only assisted teachers in structuring learning activities to achieve specific goals but helped the students become aware of the behavioral objectives they were

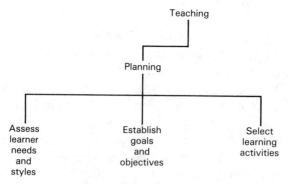

Figure  1.6
Planning Teaching Activities

expected to achieve. Taxonomies served a purpose in helping teachers evaluate goals in the cognitive domain, which tend to be in the majority, and those objectives within the affective domain, which tend to be underemphasized. Following the publishing of these taxonomies, several educators published works on writing educational objectives (Gronlund, 1978; Mager, 1962). The reader is encouraged to read these references for details.

Tyler (1949) noted that objectives should have two dimensions: 1) the behavior expected in the student as an outcome of learning; and 2) the content. An example of this type of objective would be stated as follows: "Identify the characteristics of health." The behavior expected in students is to identify the characteristics, and the content is characteristics of health. Another objective might be stated as follows: "Assess the learning needs of students." The behavior outcome is to assess, and the content is learning needs of students. The behavior in these kind of objectives is clear and the content can be identified. This way of stating objectives shows the relationship between content and process and guides the selection of learning activities involved in the behavior expected in learners.

The idea in teaching is to keep attention on the learner and to select experiences that assist learners to achieve specific objectives. The objectives are the key to what the learning experience should be. If learning is expected to take place, then objectives must be stated in terms of behavior to be expected in learners. If objectives are clearly stated then learning activities are selected to provide learners with opportunities to practice the behaviors.

**Selection of Learning Opportunities.** The guidelines for selection of experiences for learners to practice the behaviors they are expected to achieve are clearly stated objectives. Selection is also based on the teacher's assessment of learners' needs and learning styles. Some students may need more guidance and more time than others, but all should be able to achieve the objectives with adequate time, instruction, and appropriate learning resources. In a systems approach to teaching, a concept of equifinality, which states that goals can be reached from different beginnings and from different means, is demonstrated. It behooves teachers to learn about a systems approach to education, as these ideas provide flexibility in planning and selecting learning opportunities for all students based on their learning needs and learning styles.

**Implementation.** The implementation activity in teaching is brought about by student-teacher interactions and participation of both in achieving stated objectives. When students have had sufficient time and opportunities to learn the behaviors expected, whether or not these behaviors are concepts, skills, or values, evaluation determines the achievement of objectives. This phase of teaching shown in Figure 1.7 requires that teachers monitor the learning of students, guide them when necessary, and provide feedback through formative evaluations during the learning process. Student-teacher interactions are an integral part of this phase of teaching.

**Evaluation.** Teaching is directed toward specific behavioral outcomes in learners consisting of knowledge, skills, abilities, and values in the subject of the curriculum. A major outcome of teaching is that learners will achieve the objectives efficiently and effectively. A diagram of activities in evaluation is presented in Figure 1.8. Criterion measures have been identified as the standards against which behaviors are measured at the completion of a course or program. In some programs, faculty have identified critical elements that are essential in know-

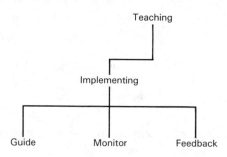

**Figure   1.7**
Implementing Teaching Activities

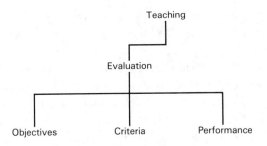

**Figure   1.8**
Evaluating Teaching Activities

ing, doing, and valuing when evaluating learners' achievements. These elements are called performance criteria whereby learners are individually evaluated. Another type of evaluation is the establishment of norms or standards which are called normative criteria and which measure achievement according to the norms of the group. The former approach to evaluation is a major element in a systems approach to instruction (Waltz et al., 1984).

### Teaching Outcomes

Measures of achievement of objectives by learners indirectly measure teaching outcomes. Teaching is guiding students through learning experiences for a purpose, to achieve specific goals. Each kind of learning requires distinct kinds of activities selected by teachers. Teaching is organized to achieve two major purposes for learners: 1) so they gain knowledge and understanding of fundamental concepts, skills, and values of the subject; and 2) so they become able to use the knowledge, skills, and values in their life and in their work. If teachers accomplish these purposes, the outcomes of teaching have been achieved. A teaching environment is another element that is essential for teachers as they facilitate learning.

### Climate for Teaching

Clearly stated goals for learning provide a major element in establishing a climate in which students have the freedom to learn and teachers have the freedom to guide the learning activities. A teaching environment that is free from bias, prejudice, and fear, in which teachers and learners have the freedom to discuss, debate, inquire, express ideas, plan, experiment, and to think, is conducive to learning and teaching. In an atmosphere of mutual respect, teachers help learners discover personal meaning and satisfaction in learning. This requires a climate in which teachers and learners form trusting relationships and are able to communicate with each other. If teaching is planning, guiding, facilitating, and evaluating, then identifying some of the characteristics of teaching should be helpful for teachers.

## Characteristics of Teaching

Some of the characteristics of teaching can describe the nature of teaching. From the theories of instruction and models of teaching, several common characteristics have been identified.

1. *Teaching is goal directed.* The teacher is responsible for establishing goals based on learner needs and styles within the objectives of the program. Goals are essential in evaluating teaching and learning outcomes.

2. *Teaching is dynamic.* Learners and teachers interact to explore goals, to agree on means to achieve goals, to explore new ideas, and to offer a variety of learning activities to help learners move toward goals.

3. *Teaching is perceiving.* Instruction involves gathering information about learners, analyzing it, interpreting it, and then verifying the accuracy of the information before making decisions.

4. *Teaching is communicating.* Communication has been identified as the information component of instruction. The use of verbal and nonverbal symbols in the teaching-learning process has been shown in studies to influence learning.

5. *Teaching is transactional.* Transactions made between teacher and learner are the valuational component of learning and relate to goals.

6. *Teaching is situational.* Activities are planned by teachers in specific situations to provide real or simulated experiences for learners to achieve goals.

7. *Teaching is a complex process.* It is characterized by choosing, planning, assessing, organizing, sequencing, facilitating, guiding, and evaluating individuals to achieve goals.

Almost all writers agree that interactions between teachers, learners, and environment influence the teaching-learning process. From the above characteristics of teaching, a definition has been formulated.

### Definition of Teaching

Teaching is a process of formulating clear objectives, assessing interests, needs, and goals of learners, setting a climate for learning, and guiding individuals through learning experiences to facilitate achievement of specific goals which results in a change in learners' knowledge, skills, and values.

### Guidelines for Teaching

Teaching helps learners see similarities and differences between present and past experiences. Information is synthesized into some kind of meaningful whole by reducing the dissonance between past and present information.

Teaching is knowing how to guide a learner through experiences that bring about motivation. Teaching that is purposeful and meaningful provides organized activities for learners to achieve goals. Teaching is helping learners use knowledge in a variety of situations. The following guidelines are offered:

1. Teaching facilitates learning when objectives are clearly stated.

2. Teaching is the selection of appropriate learning experiences and teaching strategies.

3. Teaching is a process of guiding learners through appropriate activities to achieve objectives.

4. Teaching is effective if learners achieve objectives.

5. Teaching requires evaluation and feedback.

6. Teaching provides a climate in which learners have the freedom to learn and teachers have the freedom to teach.

7. Teaching is goal directed, begins with assessment of the learners' interests, needs, and goals, and permits learners to participate in decision making.

8. Teaching is helping learners to clarify goals.

9. Teaching is seeing the world through the eyes of learners.

## A CONCEPT OF CURRICULUM

A curriculum is a subsystem within the educational system. The educational system is one kind of social system in a culture. Colleges and universities are part of the higher education system in the United States as shown in Figure 1.9.

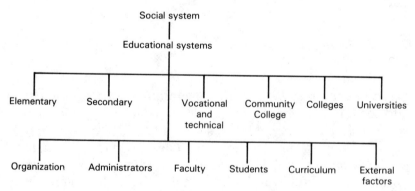

**Figure   1.9**
Education—A Social System

Educational theorizing has been going on for many years. Instructional theory is one kind of educational theory and was explored in the last section. Curriculum theory is another kind of educational theory, but the concepts of curriculum theory in the literature are not always clearly identified and defined. Many propositions have been stated about curriculum but few hypotheses have been tested in research.

### Review of Curriculum Theory

A variety of theoretical formulations have been published in the education literature. According to Beauchamp (1968), "Curriculum theory is a set of related statements that gives meaning to a school's curriculum by pointing up the relationships among its elements and by directing its development, its use, and its evaluation" (p. 67). Curriculum theory deals with those who develop, plan, implement, and evaluate the curriculum. Instructional theory, according to Beauchamp, deals with the elements related to teaching and learning. Many articles and books have been published about theories of curriculum, but research organizing basic concepts into broad generalizations is minimal. In keeping with the thesis in this book, some basic concepts have been identified from theoretical positions in education. These concepts have been organized into curriculum systems.

Three basic elements in curriculum theory were discussed by Frymier (1969). First, actors were seen as persons directly involved in curriculum, such as teachers. Second, artifacts were discussed as the content that included curriculum design. Third, operations were identified as the processes that explained the interaction of actors and artifacts. These three elements can be subsumed under Beauchamp's concepts, which were curriculum development, curriculum use, and curriculum evaluation.

A curriculum system is organized for decision making. Decisions are made about the persons who will be involved in planning and organizing the curriculum. In higher education, faculty members assume the responsibility for making decisions about the overall goals, specific objectives, and requirements for admission, retention, and graduation. Faculty members design the content in the courses and select the learning materials to be used by students. Faculty select evaluation criteria on the basis of the stated objectives.

Using the simple input-process-output model to represent an educational system, the inputs are money and resources from the public and private sectors. These inputs are transformed into buildings, books, equipment, teachers, and administrators. These transformations from inputs process people, called students, as outputs who become individuals with different kinds of education, training, and degrees.

Some of the systems literature identified several elements common in open systems. One of the first elements relates to the output of systems. For example, what is the total output of the system of education at the college and university level? It is known that the total output is not only the performance measure of the learners but the cost measured by inputs. The majority of students who graduate may be very successful in life and in their work, but what is the cost of the system? Quality of a system must be measured by some ultimate objectives, one of which is the preservation of a free society.

A second element in open systems is the environment which determines control and constraints in the system. For example, the resources available may be limited one year and increased the next year. The environment may not be under the internal control of the managers but may be determined by external forces such as state legislators or private foundations.

A third element common to open systems related to resources has been classified as human resources in the form of personnel and material resources in the form of money and equipment.

The fourth element is the structure of open systems which determines control over decision making about allocations of the resources that will be made available for the activities to be performed.

A fifth element is related to the functions to be performed to achieve the goals of the system. For example, one would identify the number of teachers required, the number of hours spent in teaching, the number of classrooms used, the type of equipment available, and the books. Any function is viewed as a critical component in the self-regulating and dynamic equilibrium of the system. A systems approach is shown in Figure 1.10.

The input into the curriculum system comes from society in the form of money from public and private sources, from the community in terms of educational needs of citizens, and from parents who pay the bills. In addition, input is provided by professionals, such as educational administrators, teachers, counselors, and professional organizations.

*Curriculum planning* requires that individuals who are responsible form a group to identify the tasks, time, and resources. In higher education the faculty in each field of study is held accountable for developing courses in the curriculum and in recommending revisions when necessary. Questions serve as guidelines for a faculty group. What are the goals to be accomplished by the curriculum? How should the faculty be organized to achieve the goals? Who will assess contemporary practices in the field of study? What are the criteria or guidelines for decision making about curriculum goals, design, implementation, and evaluation? The primary goal of the faculty is to design instruction for learning.

*Curriculum design* results in the identification of program goals from which an instructional design is derived. Specific objectives and learning activities are selected. These activities determine some of the teaching strategies. When decisions are implemented, these inputs are transformed into outputs called learning outcomes. Figure 1.11 shows the process.

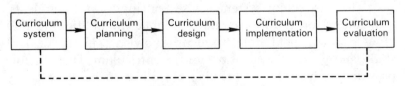

**Figure 1.10**
A Curriculum System

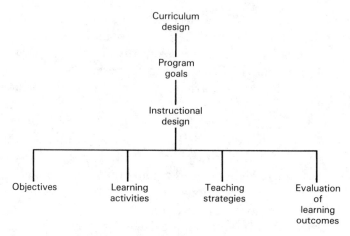

**Figure   1.11**
Curriculum Design

*Curriculum implementation* is putting into practice the re-sults of planning and designing a curriculum.

An instructional design shown in Figure 1.12 provides a specific guide to implementation of a curriculum. The specific objectives aid in selection of learning opportunities which help select teaching strategies. During the implementation phase, feedback is an important element. This requires some type of evaluation process throughout the implementation of curriculum and instruction.

*Curriculum evaluation* is built into the overall system. One evaluation model that includes evaluation in each element of developing and implementing a curriculum is called CIPP, Context, Input, Product, Process (Stufflebeam, 1971). Use of this model is described in developing and implementing a graduate program in nursing (Steele, 1978).

The curriculum system has several inputs from students, professional organizations, and the public. In addition, faculty input plays a major role based on knowledge in the field of study and previous evaluations of the curriculum. These factors provide the basis for identifying objectives to be achieved by students.

Evaluation is a kind of output of the system that tells

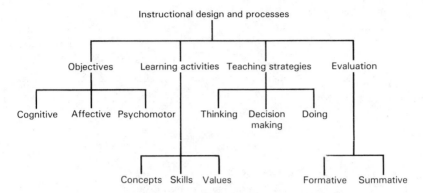

**Figure 1.12**
Instructional Design and Processes

about the systems performance and provides input into the system to set the process in motion again. A primary function of the curriculum is to help learners achieve objectives. Faculty members use formative evaluation to guide the learning process. To determine if their outcome behaviors have met performance criteria, summative evaluation methods that either observe or measure the behaviors are used. The process of summative evaluation of learners is also one method for evaluating a curriculum.

Concepts that have been used in curriculum planning and designing have been selected to provide a theoretical basis for curriculum development. Curriculum decision makers must account for the nature of knowledge in a field of study that is essential for learners entering the field, the nature of the learners, and the process of knowing. A process diagram that is useful in developing a curriculum is shown in Figure 1.13. Input into this process originates with faculty. Citizens, students, and others provide input into the process. From a synthesis of the literature, a few characteristics have been identified.

### Characteristics of a Curriculum

Curricula are designed for elementary, secondary, and higher education programs in the educational system of each state in

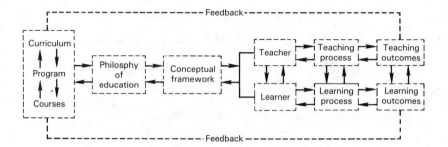

**Figure 1.13**
Curriculum Development Process

the United States. Curricula are designed for community colleges, senior colleges, and universities, and reflect liberal arts, sciences and humanities, preprofessional programs of studies, programs for occupations, and programs for professions. Faculty members in higher education have responsibility to design curricula. Faculty members serve on the policy-making committees where decisions are made about the liberal or general education components required for an undergraduate degree. Some general characteristics of a curriculum are identified that can be used irrespective of the field of study.

1. Curriculum is goal directed and prescribes the results of instruction. Curriculum decisions structure the learning outcomes of instruction, which are the means to achieve goals.

2. Curriculum is the output of the educational system and the input in the instructional system.

3. Curriculum is designed on the basis of the needs of society and the nature and needs of the individuals who will be influenced by it.

4. Curriculum plans include goals, resource materials, and learning activities, organized sequentially to provide continuity in the learning process.

5. Curriculum implementation provides for formative evaluations, feedback to learners and the curriculum system for corrective action if necessary.

6. Curriculum evaluation provides for summative evaluation of learners to determine achievement of behavior outcomes.

7. Curriculum evaluation provides feedback to decision makers about the effectiveness of the curriculum.

8. Curriculum development or revision involves a wide range of human relations.

From the concepts in curriculum theorizing and the characteristics of a curriculum, a definition is derived.

### Definition of a Curriculum

A curriculum is a systematically planned, organized, and structured program to achieve the goals of individuals and society, resulting in knowledge, skills, and values in a field of study and a commitment to protect and preserve the culture.

### Guidelines for Curriculum Development

Guidelines serve as organizing foci in developing a curriculum. The following questions have been useful in working with faculty groups to develop a curriculum.

1. What goals are to be attained by students upon graduation from a program?

2. What is the organizing focus for the program?

3. What behavior outcomes are expected in the students upon graduation?

4. What kind of learning experiences can be organized to bring about these changes in behavior?

5. How can one find out if these changes have taken place?

6. What knowledge, skills, abilities, attitudes, values, and habits are expected in students upon graduation?

7. Is there a balance in the learning experiences? Or is the content overloaded with one kind of learning?

8. What is the sequential development of the content and related learning experiences?

9. Is the curriculum organized to educate a generalist or a specialist?

When these questions are answered by faculty, a curriculum may be developed.

If the philosophy of education and psychology of learning indicate that teachers are facilitators of the learning process rather than transmitters of knowledge, controllers of learning, or directors of learners, then the curriculum reflects that learners are active participants in the learning process. This philosophical position requires that teachers grasp the process of knowing. Since teachers and learners are key inputs, processors, and outputs in the curriculum system, concepts of learning, teaching, and curriculum are essential knowledge for functioning in the role of teacher and learner.

## ROLES OF LEARNER AND TEACHER

Three major concepts have been discussed relative to curriculum and instruction. The first, learning, provided guidelines for the role of learners. The second, teaching, provided guidelines for the role of teachers. Teachers perform many functions within their role. The third, curriculum, requires knowledge about learning, learner, curriculum development, instruction, curriculum evaluation and revision.

### Role of Learner

With the current state of knowledge about how persons learn and how fast they can learn, the role of learners is an important component in the teaching-learning process. Learning is self-activity and requires involvement of each individual in the process. No one can learn for another person. In the course of growth and development, individuals recognize that learning things about their world helps them achieve goals. When goal attainment is achieved through purposeful behaviors that are learned, individuals feel rewarded and have a sense of satisfaction in being able to perform specific things. The role of learner is one of active involvement in the learning process with some input into the objectives to be achieved.

### Role of Teacher

Teachers have exhibited a variety of functions within their role. A primary function has been to guide learners through activities to achieve stated goals. In this capacity, teachers are resource persons, planners, facilitators, implementers, and evaluators. Teachers recognize learners as human beings with their individual needs, goals, interests, values, past experiences and expectations. A second function of the teacher is to evaluate learners and the curriculum. This function requires knowledge of curriculum development and instruction and evaluation of learners' performance. A third function is self-evaluation of learners' performance.

If the teacher is a critical variable in the learning process (several theories and models of teaching have indicated the influence a teacher has on learners), then what are some of the characteristics of effective teachers? Articles, conference reports and small studies of teacher effectiveness have been reported for many years. Generally, several characteristics have been identified such as intelligence, knowledge of the subject, some educational theory, interest, enthusiasm, and possesses skills in teaching.

Several problems in evaluating teaching effectiveness have been identified in the nursing literature (Stafford and Graves, 1978). Faculty members in higher education are evaluated on the basis of criteria used for other disciplines such as teaching, research and publications, and community service. In addition, nursing faculty are evaluated on both classroom teaching and clinical competence they demonstrate. A model for judging teaching effectiveness was proposed by Norman and Haumann (1978). They proposed a formal evaluation program for objective decision-making. From a review of studies related to students' perception and evaluation of teachers, twelve characteristics were identified (Kiker, 1973). The characteristics perceived to be important were professional competence, positive interpersonal relationships, ability to identify principles, availability of instructors to students, consideration of students' time, pleasant voice, and the ability to remain calm. Kiker's sample was composed of thirty undergraduate education students, thirty-seven undergraduate nursing students and thirty-six graduate nursing students. She used a questionnaire to gather information about the twelve characteristics found in the review of literature and grouped them into three categories. Six characteristics were grouped under "professional competence." Three characteristics were grouped under "relationships with students." Three characteristics were categorized under "personal attributes." Professional competence had a higher value for learners than personal characteristics. Flexibility was ranked high by both groups of nursing students who responded. Fair evaluations were placed in the top half of their rank of important characteristics in effective teachers. The graduate students in nursing valued independent thinking and learning most highly.

With the advent of computers into almost every educational system, teachers will be required to make decisions about this new tool to offer learning activities for the students of today and tomorrow. All of the technology complements and assists the human elements in the teaching role.

Although the roles of teacher and learner are distinct and different in many ways, there are some common characteristics related to education. One is shared goal setting, exploring means to achieve goals with both teacher and student working to help the students achieve the goal of learning. Another shared goal is preserving the society by learning something that prepares one for useful, constructive, happy living and working.

The two roles are paramount in the educational system. The concepts of teaching, learning, and teacher and learner are complementary and interrelated in the learning environment.

Specific elements that influence curriculum development and instruction are a philosophy of nursing education and a conceptual framework. These elements are explored in the next two chapters.

# chapter 2

# Philosophy and Nursing Education

Philosophy is one of the oldest disciplines in higher education. Historically, the subject matter has been ontology, epistemology, the study of human nature, and the study of human actions or ethics. Philosophy, literally defined, is the search for "truth." When one studies philosophy, one inquires into the nature of persons, the essence of reality, the nature of knowledge, and the source and significance of values.

One of the basic problems that philosophers have confronted for centuries has been the problem of knowledge. The great philosophers of the past were constantly searching for "truth" through thinking, discussing, and debating the ideas of their time. Most agreed that human beings have an ability to know their world and to attain some certitude about the fundamental questions in life. Two basic premises that have prevailed in philosophy are: 1) human beings have knowledge that comes from the senses; and 2) human beings have knowledge that comes from the intellect, that is, thinking and reasoning. Sense knowledge and intellectual knowledge are complementary, as sensation is a source of intellectual knowledge.

Human beings are action oriented, which implies knowledge. Ethics, a branch of philosophy, is the study of human actions. Human beings are goal oriented, which implies values. Values are learned in one's environment. Knowledge about human–environment interactions comes from a variety of sources, such as formal education, articles and books, multimedia systems, and experience. Educational systems have been established to impart knowledge and to perpetuate the values of society. The purposes of education usually flow from a philosophy of education.

Philosophies of education are accepted or rejected on their basic premises about the nature of reality, knowledge, value, and persons and translating these ideas into educational programs whose ends and means are based on reason, logic, and empirical evidence (Power, p. 261). Analysis of propositions of different philosophies of education provides teachers with knowledge rather than opinion about educational goals and the means to attain them. Since philosophy gives direction to human actions, it seems appropriate to discuss how statements of philosophy give direction in curriculum and instruction in nursing in higher education.

This chapter identifies ideas about philosophy, philosophy of education, philosophy of nursing, and philosophy of nursing education. Examples of philosophical ideas are presented. Criteria for formulating a philosophy of nursing education are suggested for faculty consideration in writing a statement of philosophy that guides curriculum and instruction in nursing in higher education.

## WHAT IS PHILOSOPHY?

Philosophy is a search for understanding the way human beings orient themselves to a personal world of reality, to the meanings found in that world, to the values held by the individual, and to the standards of behavior that guide individual choices (Kaplan, 1961). Kaplan identified four themes in world philosophies:

1. Rationality places emphasis on intellect and understanding. Knowledge is of utmost importance and is based on the use of reason.

2. Action is an essential component in the educational process, since knowledge and understanding of one's world is the guide to individual choice and action.

3. Humanism is one way of deriving a theory of human nature which is central to knowing self and others.

4. Values influence actions.

Kaplan noted that one value was identified in which all philosophies converge, and that was the value of freedom to think and to act (pp. 8-10).

Generally, philosophy in current usage centers around two broad activities: 1) a rational, critical, and logically analytic enterprise, consisting in applying criteria of consistency and coherence to concepts and to the use of language; and 2) a more speculative enterprise that attempts to provide a vision of the way things really are.

Dewey (1963) advocated that the business of education was to plan for learning activities that led to knowledge and understanding of the subject matter and the world.

Phenix (1961) noted that philosophy is a search for values that give direction for choices in one's life. When related to education, philosophy helps make choices about curricula and subject matter.

Some of the major concepts discussed in most philosophies over the past few centuries and still being debated today are: the nature of human beings, the nature of society, the nature of education, and the nature of values. Understanding these concepts provides information on decision making and standards of behavior in a society. A synthesis of the ideas from the traditional philosophic positions over the centuries is presented. The traditional philosophies have been called idealism, realism, logical positivism, Christian traditionalism, existentialism, and pragmatism. Any description of the nature of something includes the characteristics that are common to a class or group of things. The nature of something describes its essence.

### The Nature of Human Beings

Human beings are open systems in transaction with the environment. Environment includes ecosystems and space occupied by persons, animals, plants, and other objects. Transaction connotes that there is no separateness between human beings and environment.

Some of the characteristics that are common to human beings are that they are unique, holistic individuals of intrinsic worth who are capable of rational thinking and decision making. As individuals, they are sentient and social, as observed by their interactions with persons and objects in the environment. They are perceiving and reacting beings who are controlling, purposeful, action oriented, and time oriented in their behavior (King, 1981, p. 143).

Individuals have the capacity to know, think, make choices, and select alternative courses of action. Human beings have the ability through their language and other symbols to record their history and to preserve their cultures. Because of this, individual and group differences have been identified over the ages. Since individuals constitute groups and groups constitute communities which form societies, the nature of society is discussed.

### The Nature of Society

A few ideas about the nature of society in the United States are discussed. Each individual can add personal ideas to this discussion. U.S. society, through the Constitution and Bill of Rights, provides in a general way the rights and responsibilities of individuals as citizens, of individuals in relation to other citizens, and of individuals in relation to the society as a whole. This society is a microscopic open system within the world, whose main purpose has been shown to be the protection of individual freedom within the rules for protection of the common good of society and the maintenance of U.S. culture. It is a pluralistic society, dynamic in its changing technology but continuous through the preservation of some values. The freedom of individuals and of groups is protected under the judicial system. U.S. society was constructed as a democracy based on people's ability to think rationally and to make choices in the solution of individual, group, and societal problems.

Individual achievement, satisfaction, and fulfillment take place within the larger social system. In protecting rights of individuals, society also has expectations of them, that is, that they function at an optimal level in performance in their family, social, and work roles. One expectation is that individuals who can work will. Work requires some kind of education and training. Some individuals pursue educational programs that prepare them to be the thinkers, some to be the doers, some to combine thinking and doing. In this highly technical society with constant changes, individuals are often expected to continue their education as a lifelong process, while others find they must be retrained when their job becomes obsolete. This society has had a commitment to the education of its citizens. One characteristic of this society is a compulsory educational system to prepare individuals for living, working, and, recently, recreation.

## The Nature of Values

Individuals differ in their interests, needs, wants, and goals. Since each person is unique, the nature of values emanates from the nature of human beings. Values form the basis for each person's goals. If one values truth, goodness, and beauty, how will these values influence an individual's goals? If one values and respects the worth of human beings, how will this influence relationships with others? If one values knowledge and intellectual ability to solve problems, how will this influence a person's goals? If one values the personal freedom to seek knowledge, to enjoy life, to do the things that bring rewards and pleasures, then will goals be self-centered, or will these values provide a self concept that includes consideration for the welfare of others? These are just a few ideas to be considered when trying to describe the nature of values.

Values are characterized by what an individual thinks about the worth of something or its importance to achieve goals. An old cliche stated this clearly: "We value the truth, the good, and the beautiful." The truth implies a searching inquiry into the nature of things and deals with intellectual activities. The good implies standards of conduct in human behavior called moral values. The good in objects implies they are useful for achieving human goals. Anything labeled beautiful brings pleasure to human beings. Other examples of values are terms like honesty, loyalty, integrity, and the respect of one person for another.

In any decision-making situation, people are faced with questions of facts and questions of values (Simon, 1959). Values deal with standards of human conduct that have been handed down from one generation to another and are called cultural expectations. Moral concepts are a product of human experiences. Persons make choices in relation to their freedom and concomitant responsibility. Questions of facts are related to the values of science.

Bronowski (1965) and others have noted that scientists' primary purpose is to explore truth. Such a purpose implies values for the scientific process, its use in discovering truth, freedom to search for truth within the values held by scientists such as communicating your scientific findings to peers for critique. The respect of one scientist for another is shown in the way they honor colleagues for their discoveries and the way they enjoy the freedom and independence granted to a scientist. Each discipline can identify a cadre of scientists and scholars who formulate the theories of the field of study and conduct the research to test the hypotheses generated by the theories.

Values vary from person to person. When there is disagreement between two or more individuals, value conflict may occur. Each person's ideas and feelings enter into a situation. When one is pressured to make choices, intrapersonal conflict in values may occur. Values are related to learning because one's values fall within a cognitive dimension, an affective dimension, and a psychomotor dimension. For example, a scientist values thinking and independence. An actress values role playing and fantasy. A professional athlete or an Olympic runner values psychomotor skills. Goals are formulated on the basis of one's personal values. The values of society influence the educational system.

## WHAT IS A PHILOSOPHY OF EDUCATION?

Socrates, Plato, and Aristotle are noted for bringing philosophy to education under the rubric of scientific humanism. They were followed by Christian leaders, such as St. Augustine. This philosophy was called religious humanism. Through Comenius' realism in the sixteenth century and Locke's empiricism in the seventeenth century, educational philosophy made slow progress in reforming education. Rousseau caused a revolution in education thought and brought naturalism to the attention of all. Philosophy has been a dominant force in shaping educational thought for centuries. Educational philosophy gives guidance to the total educational enterprise. It deals with general principles about educational goals and the means to achieve them (Power, 1982).

Many philosophies over the centuries have influenced educational thought and policy. All have some commonalities but all reflect differences in beliefs about human beings, knowledge, society, and values.

Power (1982) has outlined clearly the philosophical principles of idealism, realism, pragmatism, and existentialism as they related to the nature of the person, of reality, of knowledge, and of value (pp. 71–152). He noted that a philosophy of education guides policy, and policy is translated into practices in the educational system (p. 20).

## The Nature of Education

The term education literally means to lead out, to bring forth, to inform, and to enlighten. Education is characterized by training the mind to think, to gain knowledge through engagement in intellectual activities, to search for truth, to disseminate knowledge to all citizens, and to encourage continuous intellectual growth of citizens.

Education is that social system within a society that provides formal programs for individuals to acquire knowledge and to develop concepts and skills to prepare them for the world of living and the world of work. Education should help individuals live a useful and happy life. Education should help persons learn how to solve problems and to cope with stress and change. Education in a technological society prepares individuals with process skills and with content in a subject of their choice so they can know and do something well.

The system of education in the United States is compulsory

through the adolescent years. The dual system, public and private, gives individuals flexibility and choice of educational environments. Also, choices are provided for pursuing particular types of educational experiences. For example, vocational and technical programs are offered in community colleges and technical institutes. Preprofessional and professional education is offered in colleges and universities. Graduate education is offered in colleges and universities.

The essence of education has been the communication of information about knowledge, skills, and values of a society. Through education, the cultural traditions of a society have been preserved. Education has provided a formal system for imparting knowledge to each succeeding generation in a society and at the same time adding new knowledge and technologies from research and development.

Education is the one facet of a society in which the primary function has been to train the minds of all citizens and to help them acquire the intellectual and practical methods to function in society. Individuals learn about the problems in life and scientific ways to solve the problems. The knowledge and skills learned can be used in living and working in society.

Education provides for intellectual, emotional, and social growth of human beings. Education demonstrates balance between freedom and individual responsibility. The ultimate goal of education is the pursuit and dissemination of truth. Commitment to lifelong learning requires continuing education for adults in a technological society. Individual goals help in making decisions about the type of education one will pursue.

Educational philosophy provides a plan for what is conceived to be the best formal education for human beings. Educational philosophy interprets and gives direction for implementation of the kind of education that will achieve individual and societal purposes. It gives precise direction to implement educational practice that is viewed to serve society best. Educational philosophy conducts investigations into the whole of the educational system, evaluates it, justifies it, or reforms its policies and practices (Power, 1982, pp. 15-16).

### Definition of Philosophy of Education

A philosophy of education shows how human reason determines the structure and functions of education in a specific society and includes philosophical assumptions that guide teaching and learning (McClellan, 1976). Generally speaking, a philosophy of education is "any reasonably coherent set of values and fundamental assumptions used as a basis for evaluation and guidance of educational practice" (Phenix, 1961, p. 4).

Since each profession is based on its own set of philosophical assumptions which flow from society, from the identified social need, and from the human beings for which the service is provided, a philosophy of nursing and nursing education is explicated.

## WHAT IS A PHILOSOPHY OF NURSING?

A philosophy of nursing includes basic premises about the nature of nursing, about the goal of nursing, about rights to health and concomitant obligations for maintaining health, and about the role of nurses in health-care systems in society.

Nursing as a recognized profession has been given a trusteeship by society. Nursing has as its focus the care of individuals and groups along with social interactions and social movements that influence health care.

Some understanding of human–environment transactions is prerequisite to understanding the nature of nursing (King, 1981). As professionals, nurses deal with the behavior of individuals and groups in potentially stressful situations relative to health and illness and help people meet their basic needs in order to perform activities of daily living. The nature of nursing is also described in terms of the functions of nurses.

Nursing is a helping profession because nurses care about and for human beings. Nursing cuts across age and socioeconomic barriers. Nurses provide a service that meets a social need. A part of this service is to give care to individuals and groups who are acutely and moderately ill and usually hospitalized. Nurses give care to individuals in the home, to those with chronic ill-nesses, and to those who need rehabilitation to help them use their potential ability to function as human beings. Nurses offer guidance to help individuals maintain health. Nurses are partners with physicians in promoting health, in preventing disease, and in managing patient care. They cooperate and collaborate with families, physicians, and allied health professionals to coordinate a plan of care for individuals (King, 1971, p. 119; King, 1976, p. 52). Nurses are recognized as an essential group in the delivery of quality health services to the public.

Nurses are expected to synthesize knowledge from natural and behavioral sciences and from nursing science and to use knowledge in making decisions to meet basic needs of individuals that are immediate in nursing situations. Nurses are required to plan with individuals to help them learn ways to cope with ill-ness and health problems in the future and to adjust to changes in health states.

> Nurses play strategic roles in the process of human growth and de-velopment and in helping individuals cope with disturbances in their health. They have an essential role in community planning for the delivery of health services to the public. As professionals, nurses deal with behavior of individuals and groups in potentially stressful situa-tions, pertaining to health, illness, and crises, and help people cope with changes in daily activities (King, 1981, p. 13)

> Nursing is perceiving, thinking, relating, judging, and acting vis-a-vis the behavior of individuals who come to a nursing situation. A nurs-ing situation is the immediate environment, spatial and temporal reality, in which nurse and client establish a relationship to cope with health states and adjust to changes in activities of daily living if the situation demands adjustment (King, 1981, p. 2).

> Nursing is defined as a process of action, reaction and interaction whereby nurse and client share information about their perceptions in the nursing situation. Through purposeful communications they identify specific goals, problems or concerns. They explore means to achieve a goal and agree to means to do this. When clients par-ticipate in goal setting with professionals, they interact with nurses to move toward goal attainment in most situations (King, 1981, p. 2).

Nurses coordinate the delivery of health care. The expanded role of nurses from primarily care of the sick to maintenance and restoration of health provides additional services related to health. Knowledge of human behavior is essential to understand the nature of nursing, whose focus is human–environment transactions.

An essential part of an educational program that prepares young men and women to become professional practitioners is assistance for them as students to acquire the ways of searching for knowledge and for using knowledge in the practice of nursing. The basis for the practice of professional nursing is knowledge; the activity is guided by the intellect, and its intellectual activity is applied in the practical realm. Nurses are expected to possess intellectual skills, interpersonal skills, and technical skills. The searching inquiry into the nature of nursing as learners helps to establish the foundations for practice upon graduation, and for continuous learning throughout life. A philosophy of nursing gives direction to a philosophy of nursing education.

## WHAT IS A PHILOSOPHY OF NURSING EDUCATION?

In the early part of the twentieth century, three volumes were published to serve as guides for curriculum development in schools of nursing (National League for Nursing Education, 1917, 1927, 1937). Analysis of curriculum surveys and studies in nursing education and the need for explicating a philosophy of nursing education as an essential component for curriculum development was suggested in the third curriculum guide (NLNE, 1937).

Isabel Maitland Stewart directed the 1937 curriculum study and involved many nurses throughout the United States. She noted that "a philosophy of education is a characteristic attitude toward education and its problems with special reference to the purposes and goals to be achieved and the methods by which they are to be reached" (p. 14). This third curriculum study indicated that a statement of a philosophy of education and of the purpose for a school of nursing were the basis for a quality curriculum. Stewart stated that "only by agreeing to a common philosophy and aim is it possible to have anything like unity and consistency in an education program" (p. 14). She also noted,

> Some kind of philosophy lies back of every curriculum. It may not be explicitly stated nor consistent but it nevertheless determines the type of subject matter selected, the methods of instruction used, and the way in which the whole program is constructed and operated (p. 15).

The studies reported before and after 1937 have implied the need to provide unity and consistency in the philosophy, purpose and objectives of a program (Goldmark, 1923; Committee on Grading of Nursing Schools, 1928, 1934; Brown, 1948; West and Hawkins, 1950; Montag, 1951, 1959; Bridgman, 1953; Lambertson, 1958; Lysaught, 1970).

Several articles and studies have been selected from the literature to indicate a trend toward more nurses writing about a philosophy of nursing and nursing education. As the reader reviews the literature, you will find many sources of ideas that are useful in trying to write your philosophy of nursing education.

Personal beliefs of individual nurses that reflect their philosophy have been published for many years (Goodrich, 1929; Taylor, 1934; Heidgerken, 1959; Clemence, 1962; Hall, 1964). Several philosophical assumptions from idealism, realism, experimentalism, neoThomism, and existentialism were suggested as one approach to identify an "eclectic philosophy of nursing education" (Treece, 1974). Some nurses stated that a philosophy should focus on the nature of the "whole person" and the nature of learning. Others indicated that philosophical considerations should be given to the nature of the adult learner, purposes for educational activities that influence cognitive and affective growth of an individual, and active participation of learners and consumers in making decisions about their experiences (Croll, 1977; Tribbles, 1977; King, 1981).

Several nurses have related the philosophic themes of Marcel and Buber, contemporary existential philosophers, to current concepts in nursing, such as patient centered nursing care, student centered learning, commitment to care of individuals (Black, 1964; Ferlic, 1968; Zasowska, 1974; Ulsafer, 1976; Patterson and Zderad, 1976). These authors generally agreed that professional nurses demonstrated commitment because of involvement with patients/clients through their caring and love and their giving and receiving.

Several philosophical themes of Buber and Marcel were analyzed by Nelson (1977). Commitment, presence, existence, and intersubjectivity were identified as relevant themes for nursing. She suggested that nurse educators "give serious consideration to the integration of existentialism as a humanistic philosophic base which can help to illuminate and clarify nursing practice" (Nelson, 1977, p. 198).

A national survey of philosophies of nursing education has shown some differences and similarities in use of terms in statements of philosophies of nursing education (King, 1984). A random sample of nursing programs, stratified by four regions of the United States and by three types of programs, diploma, associate degree, and baccalaureate, was selected from the 1979 published list of NLN accredited schools. A primary purpose of the study was to identify similarities and differences in the terms used in statements of philosophies of nursing education. A category system of terms had been identified prior to analyzing the philosophy statements.

The findings of the study indicated that there were statistically significant differences in major terms used in the three types of programs. However, terms which seemed common to all programs were nursing, environment, and interpersonal relations. The major terms identified in this study were human being, role, perception, interpersonal relations, social systems, health, environment, nursing, and God. The unit of analysis chosen was the word because words used by individuals are symbolic representations of beliefs. Words used in statements of philosophies of nursing education identify concepts that faculty believe are relevant for their types of program.

This national survey had implications for faculty groups

that write the future statements of philosophies for their educational programs. Analysis of philosophies indicated that some faculty groups used terms and sentences that described the nature of human beings, the nature of learners, and the nature of nursing, while other statements were concrete and factual and indicated purpose rather than philosophy.

One recommendation from this study was a need to identify a set of guidelines for writing a philosophy of nursing education. These guidelines can provide for unity and consistency in philosophic pronouncements and are stated here.

### Guidelines for Formulating a Philosophy

The following ideas are offered to provide some structure for faculty groups to write a philosophy for a nursing curriculum:

1. Statements about the nature of nursing as it relates to human beings, to health, to human rights to health, human obligations for health, and the role of nurses in health care systems in this society. For example, human beings are time oriented, react as total persons, and have rights to quality care.

2. Statements about the nature of learning, of teaching, and of education for the practice of nursing as professionals. Opportunities are provided for students to have freedom to learn. Teachers have a responsibility to provide a climate for learning.

3. Statements about professional values in nursing, such as, nurses are accountable first to the clients they serve and then to the profession. Another example is that individuals have the right to accept or reject health care.

Statements of philosophical assumptions emanating from the above guidelines will assist faculty members in their discussion of beliefs about nursing education.

Nursing education prepares individuals for something they

know well and can do well. Education for nursing recognizes each person as a human being and a social being and so prepares individuals intellectually and socially. Individuals have rights, duties, and obligations related to self, to others, and to society. Recognition is given to the fact that individuals have been a part of education beginning with the family and progressing in formal programs in schools and colleges. In addition, nursing education is responsible for inculcating the values of the profession within an educational program. Nursing education recognizes the right of the learners to have the freedom to learn and the teachers to have the freedom to teach.

An assumption is made that nursing education takes place in an institution of higher education whose primary purpose is education for professions and education for highly skilled technicians. Community colleges are a part of the system of higher education in most states. A philosophy of nursing education recognizes learners with individual differences in abilities and in learning styles, the society in which learners are citizens, and the occupations or professions to which the learners aspire.

In summary, philosophy deals with questions whose answers depend on philosophical knowledge, such as who is being educated, what are the goals, and what are the means to achieve the goals. Philosophical principles are used to formulate educational policy, and policy is used to organize who shall be taught, what shall be taught, and what will be the means used to achieve the goals. These principles bring philosophy to a practical level of teaching and learning in a formal curriculum within an educational system in a society. The following criteria are suggested for use in stating a philosophy of nursing education:

1.  Every individual is a social being with rights, duties, and obligations.

2.  Education provides for continuing development of the intellectual, emotional, and social dimensions in learners resulting in an individual who thinks, judges, and acts consistently in accordance with reason.

3. Every profession has a system of values exhibited by its members.

4. Nursing is an essential social service and education is a continuous, lifelong process.

5. Cognitive, affective, and psychomotor behaviors are recognized as the domains of learning.

These criteria and the guidelines from the national survey of philosophies of nursing education provided the basis for an example of a statement of a philosophy of nursing education that may guide curriculum and instruction in nursing in higher education.

## A PHILOSOPHY OF NURSING EDUCATION

The philosophical assumptions are categorized under the nature of human beings, society, health care delivery systems, nursing, higher education, learning, teaching, and nursing education. Several ideas are presented under each of these categories as examples of faculty beliefs.

### Nature of Human Beings

Human beings are open systems in continuous transactions with the environment. Individuals act both individually and as members of various groups, such as the family, community, and society. Human beings are unique, holistic persons of intrinsic worth who are capable of sensing, relating, communicating, thinking, and making decisions. Individuals act in a purposeful manner based on their perceptions, background of experiences, interests, and goals.

### Nature of Society

U.S. society is pluralistic and offers freedom for individuals under the Constitution. An implicit assumption is that society accepts the fact that health or optimum wellness is both a right and a responsibility of individual members. Society provides for health-care delivery systems to care for those members who are ill, who have a disease, and who are handicapped. Emphasis on health has been promoted recently.

### Nature of Health Care Delivery Systems

Health care in the United States has become one of the largest industries in the 1980's. The most recent systems of care are described as primary, secondary, and tertiary. Ethical issues have been identified that relate to health care of individuals and high technology available in treatment and therapy. Society assumes that health professionals will preserve the dignity of human beings in treatment and care and help people maintain a level of wellness for them to function in their roles in society. Health professionals are expected to use knowledge and skills to assist individuals in need of care and to help individuals maintain dignity during terminal illness.

### Health

Health has a high priority in our society. The World Health Organization (WHO) has worked also to place health high in the value systems of many nations. Health relates to the way individuals cope with the stresses of growth and development while functioning in a culture in which they were born and to which they attempt to conform (King, 1971, p. 67). Health is defined as

> dynamic life experiences of a human being, which implies continuous adjustment to stressors in the internal and external environment through optimum use of one's resources to achieve maximum potential for daily living (King, 1981, p. 5).

Health practices are learned in the family with continuation of this learning in schools, in groups and in the community (Clements and Roberts, 1983).

## Nature of Nursing

The goal of nursing is to help persons maintain their health so they can function at an optimum level in their social roles. "The domain of nursing includes promotion of health, maintenance and restoration of health, care of the sick and injured and care of the dying" (King, 1981, p. 4). Nursing is perceiving, thinking, relating, judging, acting, interacting, and transacting with individuals who come to a nursing situation.

> A nursing situation is the immediate environment, spatial and temporal reality, in which nurse and client establish a relationship to cope with health states and adjust to changes in activities of daily living if the situation demands adjustment (King, 1981, p. 4).

Nursing is defined as "a process of action, reaction, and interaction whereby nurse and client share information about their perceptions in a nursing situation" (King, 1981, p. 2). Through purposeful communication they identify specific goals, problems, or concerns. They explore means to achieve a goal and agree to means to use to reach the goal. When clients participate in goal setting with professionals, they interact with nurses to move toward goal attainment in most situations. Professional nursing involves the use of knowledge and the use of self in assessing, planning, diagnosing, goal setting, implementing, and evaluating nursing care to meet the needs of individuals and groups. Professional nursing, through the actions of its members, demonstrates accountability and responsibility to society. The functions of professional nursing are interdependent and collaborative with other health professionals in order to meet a societal mandate for quality health care.

### Nature of Higher Education

Higher education is a formal educational system, publicly and privately controlled, given a mandate by society to prepare individuals to live and work in society and to preserve the democratic ideals of a free society. This formal system of education provides programs in vocational fields, in semi-professional and technical fields, in liberal and professional education. This system recognizes individual differences in learners and offers programs to facilitate learning to achieve maximum human potential.

### Nature of Learning

Learning is a dynamic and lifelong process of change whereby individuals cope with living and working in society. Learning is an individualized experience and involves several major variables. These variables are clearly stated goals, appropriate learning activities, teacher guidance, willingness of learner to perform activities essential to achieve objectives. Learning is self-activity, because no one can learn for another individual. Learning is involvement of individuals through their perceptual experiences to react to stimuli in the environment and to form concepts about reality. Learning is dynamic, because each new experience increases information about reality. Learning is goal oriented in that when individuals value something, they tend to learn what will help them achieve a goal. Learning is a self-regulating process in that feedback from the environment influences inputs and outputs such as learning outcomes. Reinforcement through feedback verifies a person's reality and gives satisfaction in attainment of goals. Learning is characterized by thinking and judging events, persons, and things in the environment. Each individual develops, grows, and learns as a whole person. Each individual has a unique learning style and personal goals and learns at his or her own pace. Each learner brings to an educational program his or her own background of experiences which account for some of the individual differences.

## Nature of Teaching

Teaching is planning, implementing, and evaluating learning. Teaching is providing a climate conducive to individual growth and freedom to inquire into the nature of the environment. Teaching is goal directed based on the learner's interests and learning style. Teaching is guiding learners through communications to attain information. Teaching is a complex process characterized by choosing, planning, assessing, organizing, sequencing, facilitating, guiding, and evaluating individuals to achieve goals. Teaching is a process of formulating clear objectives, assessing the interests, needs, and goals of learners, setting a climate for learning, guiding individuals through learning experiences, and facilitating achievement of specific goals which result in change in learners' knowledge, skills, and values.

## Nature of Nursing Education

A philosophy of nursing education states assumptions about the nature of human beings interacting with environment, the purpose of nursing, values and norms of the profession, assumptions about learning, and how human reason determines the structure and functions of education for professional nursing in society (King, 1980). An educational program that aims to prepare individuals to become professional nurses is organized so the individuals admitted are active participants in the experiences and learn how to think, make decisions, and act consistently and reasonably as members of a profession and of a democratic society (King, 1980). The educative process takes place in an educational institution through planned and purposeful learning experiences based on clearly stated objectives, guided by qualified faculty members who recognize and accept individual differences in learners. Faculty members also recognize their role and responsibilities to guide learners on the basis of identified learning background and styles. The ideas presented here are examples of the kind of statements faculty groups may consider as they develop and or revise the philosophy that guides the curriculum. A philosophy gives faculty direction in formulating a conceptual framework. A conceptual framework provides structure for developing curricula and designing instruction.

# chapter 3

# Structure for Curriculum Design

A conceptual framework provides structure for a curriculum. Why does a curriculum need structure? Several reasons have been discussed and the most obvious one is that facts are too numerous to teach and to learn and facts are easily forgotten unless used. Knowledge in every field is so vast that it is difficult for teachers to select what is essential to be learned in any field of study.

*What purpose does a conceptual framework serve in developing a curriculum in nursing in higher education?* A framework helps faculty to identify and develop relevant concepts that serve as the knowledge base for professional nursing practice. A framework organizes relevant dimensions of the course of studies. When the major concepts are identified in a curriculum, students develop the concepts rather than memorize facts. Conceptual knowledge is retained for recall at a later time. As new knowledge becomes available it can be categorized within concepts learned. New knowledge refines the framework. General *functions of a conceptual framework* are:

1.  To provide a way to organize a multitude of facts into meaningful wholes, e.g. health, communication, and daily activities.

2.  To provide a common theoretical basis for communications and relationships in a field of study.

3.  To direct attention to processes and relationships which are a built-in guarantee for continued learning.

4.  To guide you to look for specific facts.

5.  To provide a way to order knowledge for use in a variety of settings.

Concepts of the framework are the organizing dimensions. Specifically, the *functions of a conceptual framework for nursing* are:

1.  To provide a basic organizing focus for the domain of nursing which structures curricula.

2. To provide a system for classifying the knowledge, skills, and values of the field of nursing.

3. To provide a way of ordering facts into a system that organizes subject matter into a whole system.

4. To show relationships in the content and processes essential for nursing.

The *functions of a conceptual framework for curriculum development* provide structure:

1. To identify goals.

2. To show behavioral objectives and content organization in harmony with the program's philosophy.

3. To guide the development of instructional materials.

4. To determine the evaluation design.

A conceptual *framework for major content elements* provides structure:

1. To select concepts.

2. To select relevant skills, such as problem solving, communication, interview, and technical assessment.

3. To promulgate the values of the profession, such as the right to privacy, the right to information about what is happening about treatments, tests, and drugs, and the right to participate in decisions about one's life and health.

4. To demonstrate application of knowledge and use of skills and values in nursing situations.

A conceptual framework shown in Figure 3.1 will be used to discuss these functions (King, 1981, p. 11).

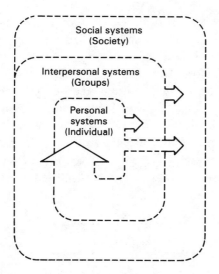

**Figure 3.1**
Dynamic Interacting Systems (From: I.M. King,
*A Theory for Nursing: Concepts, Process, and
Systems*. New York: John Wiley, 1981, p. 11.)

## KING'S CONCEPTUAL FRAMEWORK

King's systems framework guides teachers to select essential
knowledge, skills, and values of the nursing profession. The
American Nurses Association (ANA) Code for nurses, the ANA
standards for nursing practice, and the state law that licenses
nurses provide essential legal and ethical information to be
learned. Nursing process is the standard method for applying
the scientific method in a humanistic way in nursing situations
(Yura and Walsh, 1983). When this framework is used to develop
a curriculum, students learn about the major concepts of social
systems which help them understand the environment and the
health-care systems in which they will function after graduation.
Social systems represent the external environment in which

individuals make transactions to achieve goals. The major curriculum elements are diagrammed in Figure 3.2.

The concepts listed horizontally are a part of each course in the nursing major. They provide a major focus for gaining knowledge and for applying knowledge in nursing situations related to human beings, family, health, and roles of consumers and health-care providers in health-care systems. The concepts listed vertically are a part of each course in the nursing major. They provide a major focus related to human beings' perceptions, communication, interaction within organizations, and use

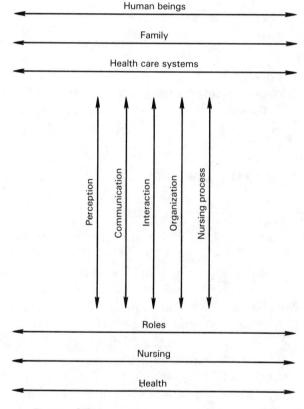

**Figure 3.2**
Major Curriculum Concepts as Organizing Elements

of the nursing process. These horizontal and vertical concepts are the organizing elements for content.

In addition, subconcepts within each of the three dynamic interacting systems of the conceptual framework are identified as substantive content. In using a general systems conceptual framework to develop a curriculum, the following basic premises and concepts are noted in Figure 3.3.

1. The focus for nursing is individuals transacting with environments.

2. The goal for nursing is health; i.e., promotion of health; preservation of health; prevention of disease, illness, and disability; care for individuals with illness, disease, and disability to help them achieve a state of

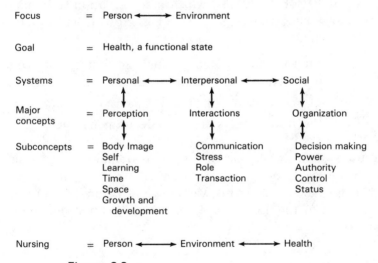

**Figure 3.3**

General Systems Conceptual Framework (From: I.M. King, "How does the conceptual framework provide structure for the curriculum?" in *Curriculum Process for Developing or Revising Baccalaureate Nursing Programs*. New York: National League for Nursing, 1978, p. 31.)

health in which they can function in their usual roles; and assistance to persons so they can die with dignity.

3. The dynamic interacting systems in Figure 3.1 are:

   a. Personal systems, which are individuals.

   b. Interpersonal systems, which are dyads, triads, small and large groups.

   c. Social systems, which are the groups that form to achieve specific purposes with society, such as the family, the school, the hospital, industry, and the church.

4. The major concepts within the three interacting systems that are essential content for nursing are:

   a. Personal systems, which are perception, self, body image, time, space, learning, growth, and development.

   b. Interpersonal systems, which are interaction, communication, transaction, stress, and role.

   c. Social systems, which are organization, power, authority control, status, and decision making.

Because systems have goals, this systems framework has health for individuals, groups and society as its goal. This framework with major and subconcepts was shown in Figure 3.3. Further explanation of the use of this framework is given in subsequent chapters.

### What is the Purpose of a Conceptual Framework?

A framework provides structure for a field of study, introduces learners to basic theoretical knowledge and to ways of inductive and deductive thinking. It helps them value their own subjective thinking and feelings.

Various methods of studying nursing phenomena are used in developing concepts. One method was demonstrated in the approach used in Chapter 1 by the author to develop the concepts presented. The way concepts from the framework were identified as substantive content in the previous section has been a problem in some faculty groups. The question most often asked is, "How do you identify content from a conceptual framework?" My response is that the concepts of the framework represent the knowledge one believes is essential for nurses to learn or faculty would not have adopted the particular framework.

The next question asked is, "How do you teach a concept to students?" My response is, "You don't teach a concept; you help students develop their own concepts by sharing your concept of the subject matter with them and guiding them in developing their own knowledge." For example, in my conceptual framework, the concepts are the specific content to be learned and this represents theoretical knowledge if one develops each concept. This theoretical knowledge is used by students when teachers plan learning experiences for them in concrete nursing situations. An example may clarify these statements. First, in my framework, health is the goal of the nursing system and is a major concept to be learned. This concept is developed in detail in later chapters. The major concepts and subconcepts of the personal systems are perception, self, body image, learning, time, space, growth, and development, and these provide substantive content to be learned. Interpersonal systems concepts are interactions, communication, stress, role, and transactions. Organization, power, authority, control, status, and decision making are essential content to be learned within social systems.

In planning the sequence of courses, primary emphasis is placed on learning about individuals. Experiences are planned for students to use that knowledge in working with all age groups relative to activities of daily living as the focus for a functional state of health. As students move from one course to another they expand their knowledge of each of these concepts and add knowledge about family and health-care systems.

These concepts also help to identify the skills as content. For example, if one is to assess a state of health, then a health assessment is performed. This requires intellectual skills and psychomotor skills until one becomes proficient in this technical skill. Measurement skills of vital signs are another example and this content comes from the major concepts of the framework. As students move through the curriculum, they make decisions in health-care systems. They have experiences in observing the use and misuse of power and authority in an organization. They recognize control in their own behavior and that of others.

The concepts of the framework are the content. This content is identified in each nursing course and learned as theoretical knowledge. A practicum course that accompanies a theory course provides selected experiences for students to use the knowledge beginning with experiences with relatively normal human beings, such as well child clinics, residents in nursing homes, children in the school system, and adults in industry and business. Then the knowledge can be used in experiences with individuals who have an interference in their ability to function in their usual roles and enter a health-care system for assistance. If students are expected to use their knowledge from the prerequisite science courses of physiology, biochemistry, and microbiology, they develop a concept of a person interacting with environment. They are able to relate this knowledge to concrete nursing situations with faculty guidance and support in the learning process. Professional values are taught as content beginning with the Code for Nurses of the ANA.

Human beings function in social systems, such as in the family, in work situations, in church, and in recreational activities, through interactions with others in terms of their perceptions and goals which influence their life and health. Professional persons have specialized knowledge, skills, and professional values in addition to personal needs, goals, and perceptions. In nursing, a process of interaction that leads to transactions helps nurses give effective nursing care in a variety of nursing situations. Several processes that are essential content in nursing are shown in Figure 3.4.

A conceptual framework produces economy in thought

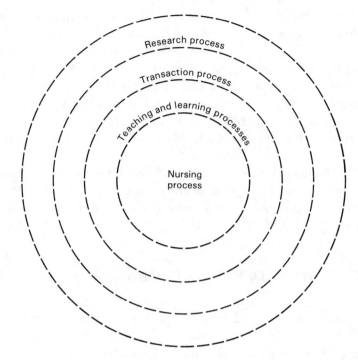

**Figure 3.4**
Process as Content

and brings order to disconnected ideas. Concepts give students freedom to explore ideas and to move forward at their own rate of speed in learning because they are not hindered by a teacher's demand to memorize facts. They are building concepts from multiple experiences with concrete facts.

A complex society with a vast accumulation of knowledge requires curricula that present the structure of knowledge in a field. Structure includes identification of essential concepts, skills, and values and organization of these elements into a framework. The concepts of the framework provide categories within which substantive facts can be selected for teaching.

In a study of fifty baccalaureate programs in 1972–73 accredited by the National League for Nursing, four common concepts were identified in all the conceptual frameworks for curricula (Torres and Yura, 1974). These concepts were human beings, health, society, and nursing. These same concepts were identified as part of a conceptual framework designed in 1971 (King, 1971). Recently, Fawcett (1984) stated that "the central concepts of the discipline of nursing are person, environment, health and nursing," since agreement comes from the nursing literature (p. 5). A national survey of philosophies of nursing education recommended the concepts of person, role, health, and society for the paradigm for professional nursing (King, 1984).

A framework gives direction to faculty to identify objectives, instructional design, and evaluation. Structure provides a systematic and consistent way of ordering concepts, skills, and values to be learned by students.

## GUIDELINES FOR A CONCEPTUAL FRAMEWORK

Guidelines are proposed here for faculty members to consider when formulating a conceptual framework for developing a curriculum. Answers to these questions not only provide a conceptual framework but can be used to evaluate a framework already in use.

1. What are the goals for professional nursing, for technical nursing, and for continuing education for nursing?

2. What knowledge is essential for a nurse to provide professional nursing care for consumers?

3. What skills are essential for professional nursing and for technical nursing?

4. What professional values are held by nurses and the profession?

5. Where do nurses perform their functions?

6. Who defines the functions of professional nurses and of technical nurses?

7. For whom do nurses provide a social service called nursing?

When the above questions have been answered to the satisfaction of the faculty group, a conceptual framework can be formulated and evaluated.

## A SUMMARY OF THE THEORETICAL BASIS

From a review of concepts from traditional schools of thought in learning, a systems view of learning, a concept of curriculum and the role of teacher and learner, a systems approach has been proposed as a basic theoretical framework for developing curricula and planning instruction.

This framework has organized concepts from learning theories into a new kind of relationship. A systems approach to learning is presented along with a few basic assumptions. First, human beings are open systems in continuous interaction with their environment. Second, the educational system within which human beings learn about their environment is an open system which is influenced by external and internal environmental factors. The educational system is one type of social system within which human beings learn in the process of growth and development. It is recognized that many social systems, such as the family, religious systems, and community groups, have some influence on learning. The educational system is established as a formal system within society to provide equality of educational opportunities for all citizens. Recognition of the background of experiences in a variety of social systems prior to individuals entering the formal educational system is essential in planning a curriculum.

The nature of the educational goal determines the teaching activities and the learning experiences that are essential to help learners achieve goals. Teachers must be prepared to develop curricula and select learning experiences for students to help them learn how to think. This is a relevant process in cognitive growth of individuals that will prepare them to meet the challenge of continuous changes in the future. The tools to think give individuals some personal control in decision making in their environment.

Educational programs are planned and implemented to prepare individuals for living in society. Professional education programs prepare individuals to function in society as professionals. This is based on an assumption that the professionals know how one can develop curricula, admit students to pass through a program, and evaluate them as having gained knowledge, skills, and values essential for a professional person.

Knowledge of learning, teaching, curriculum, role of teacher and learner, a philosophy of nursing education, and a conceptual framework is essential for individuals to develop a curriculum for an educational program. In addition, this theoretical background is essential for designing instruction, which is the core of the curriculum. The ideas presented in Part I are used in examples of curriculum and instruction in Part II designed to prepare nurses for the profession and occupation of nursing.

## REFERENCES FOR PART I

American Nurses Association. *Code for Nurses*. Kansas City, Mo.: American Nurses Association, 1976.

American Nurses Association. *Standards for Nursing Practice*. Kansas City, Mo.: American Nurses Association, 1973.

Ashby, W. Ross. *An Introduction to Cybernetics*. New York: John Wiley and Sons, 1966.

Austin, E. K. *Guidelines for the Development of Continuing Education Offerings for Nurses*. New York: Appleton-Century-Crofts, 1981.

Ausubel, D.P., *The Psychology of Meaningful Verbal Learning*. New York: Grune and Stratton, 1963.

Banathy, B.H. *Instructional Systems.* Palo Alto, Ca.: Fearon Publishers, 1968.

Beauchamp, George A. *Curriculum Theory.* 2nd ed. Wilmette, Ill.: The Kagg Press, 1968.

Bellack, Arno, et al. *The Language of the Classroom.* New York: Teachers College Press, 1963.

Bevis, E.O. *Curriculum Building in Nursing: A Process.* St. Louis: C.V. Mosby Co., 1978.

Biehler, R.F. *Psychology Applied to Teaching.* Boston: Houghton Mifflin, 1978.

Black, Sr. K. "An existential model for psychiatric nursing." *Perspectives in Psychiatric Care.* 6 (1968):174–184.

Block, James H., ed. *Mastery Learning—Theory and Practice.* New York: Holt, Rinehart and Winston, 1971.

Bloom, Benjamin S., et al. *Taxonomy of Education Objectives. Handbook I: The Cognitive Domain.* New York: David McKay Co., 1956.

Bloom, B.S.; Hastings, J.T.; and Madaus, G.F. *Handbook on Formative and Summative Evaluation of Student Learning.* New York: McGraw Hill Book Company, 1971.

Bloom, Benjamin S., et al. *Mastery Learning: Theory and Practice.* New York: Holt, Rinehart and Winston, 1971.

Bloom, Benjamin S. *Human Characteristics and School Learning.* New York: McGraw-Hill, 1976.

Bloom, Benjamin S.; Madaus, G.F.; and Hastings, J.T. *Evaluation to Improve Learning.* New York: McGraw-Hill, 1981.

Bogdan, Robert, and Taylor, Steven J. *Introduction to Qualitative Research Methods.* New York: John Wiley & Sons, 1975.

Bridgman, M. *Collegiate Education for Nursing.* New York: Russell Sage Foundation, 1953.

Bronowski, J. *Science and Human Values.* 2nd ed., rev. New York: Harper & Row, 1965.

Brown, E.L. *Nurses for the Future.* New York: Russell Sage Foundation, 1948.

Bruner, Jerome S. *The Process of Education.* New York: Vintage Books, 1960.

Bruner, Jerome S.; Goodnow, J.; and Austin, G. *A Study of Thinking.* New York: John Wiley & Sons, 1962.

Bruner, Jerome S. *Toward a Theory of Instruction.* New York: W.W. Norton, 1966.

Bruyn, Severyn T. *The Human Perspective in Sociology: The Methodology of Participant Observation.* Englewood Cliffs, N.J.: Prentice-Hall, 1966.

Carroll, J.B. "A model of school learning." *Teachers College Record* 64 (1963):723–33.

Churchman, C. West. *The Systems Approach.* New York: Dell, 1968.

Clements, I. and Roberts, F. *Family Health: A Theoretical Approach to Nursing Care.* New York: John Wiley & Sons, 1983.

Committee on Grading of Nursing Schools. *Nursing Schools Today and Tomorrow.* New York Committee, 1934.

Conley, Virginia C. *Curriculum and Instruction in Nursing.* Boston: Little, Brown, 1973.

Croll, K. "Philosophical Consideration for Inservice Education." *Journal of Continuing Education for Nursing* 8 (1977): 24–26.

Daubenmire, M.J., Searles, G.S., and Ashton, C.A. "A methodological framework to study nurse-patient communication." *Nursing Research.* 27, 5 (1978):304–310.

Davies, I.K. *Competency Based Learning: Technology, Management and Design.* New York: McGraw-Hill, 1973.

DeCecco, J.F., and Crawford, W.K. *The Psychology of Learning and Instruction.* 2nd ed. Englewood Cliffs, N.J.: Prentice-Hall, 1974.

Dewey, J. *Experience and Education.* New York: Collier Books Edition, 1963.

Eggan, P.D.; Kauchak, D.P.; and Harder, R.J. *Strategies for Teachers.* Englewood Cliffs, N.J.: Prentice-Hall, 1979.

Fawcett, J. *Analysis and Evaluation of Conceptual Models for Nursing.* Philadelphia: F.A. Davis, 1984.

Ferlic, A. "Existential Approach to Nursing." *Nursing Outlook.* 16 (1968):30–33.

Flanders, Ned A. "Interaction Analysis." In *Conceptual Models in Teacher Education,* edited by John R. Verduin, Jr. Washington, D.C.: AACTE, 1967.

Fraenkel, Jack R. *How to Teach About Values: An Analytic Approach.* Englewood Cliffs, N.J.: Prentice-Hall, 1977.

Frymier, J.R. *Fostering Educational Change.* Columbus, Oh.: Merrill Publishing Company, 1969.

Gage, N. *National Conference on Studies in Teaching.* U.S.D.H. E.W., National Institute of Education, 1975.

Gagne, Robert M. *Essentials of Learning for Instruction.* New York: Holt, Rinehart and Winston, 1975.

Gagne, Robert M. *The Conditions of Learning.* 3rd ed. New York: Holt, Rinehart and Winston, 1977.

Gagne, Robert M., and Briggs, L.J. *Principles of Instructional Design.* 2nd ed. New York: Holt, Rinehart and Winston, 1978.

Giroux, H.A.; Penna, A.N.; and Pinar, W.F. *Curriculum and Instruction.* Berkeley, Ca.: McCutchan, 1981.

Goodrich, A., "The nurse as interpreter of life." *American Journal of Nursing.* 29,4 (1929):427–428.

Goldmark, J., ed., *Nursing and Nursing Education in the United States.* New York: Macmillan, 1923.

Gronlund, N.E. *Stating Objectives for Classroom Instruction.* New York: Macmillan, 1978.

Gronlund, N.E. *Measurement and Evaluation in Teaching.* 4th ed. New York: Macmillan, 1981.

Hall, L. "Nursing—What is It?" *Canadian Nurse.* 60 (1964): 150–154.

Harrow, A.J. *A Taxonomy of the Psychomotor Domain.* New York: David McKay, 1972.

Heidergerken, L. "Some Problems in Modern Nursing." *Nursing Outlook.* 7 (1969):394–397.

Hickey, Albert E., and Newton, John M. "Logical Structure of Teaching." In *Conceptual Models in Teacher Education,* edited by John R. Verduin, Jr. Washington, D.C.: AACTE, 1967.

Hilgard, E.R., and Bower, G.H. *Theories of Learning.* 4th ed. New York: Appleton-Century-Croft, 1974.

Hill, J.E., and Kerber, A. *Models, Methods and Analytical Procedures in Education Research.* Detroit, Mich.: Wayne State University Press, 1967.

Hill, Winifred. *Learning.* New York: Harper & Row, 1977.

Huckabay, L.M. *Conditions of Learning and Instruction in Nursing.* St. Louis: C.V. Mosby, 1980.

Jones, A.S.; Bagfood, L.W.; and Wallen, E.A. *Strategies for Teaching.* Metuchen, N.J.: Scarecrow Press, Inc., 1979.

Joyce, Bruce, and Weil, Marsha. *Models of Teaching.* Englewood Cliffs, N.J.: Prentice-Hall, 1972.

Kaplan, Abraham. *The New World of Philosophy.* New York: Vintage Books, 1961.

Kiker, Myrlene. "Characteristics of the Effective Teacher." *Nursing Outlook.* 21 (1973):721–23.

King, I.M. *Toward a Theory for Nursing.* New York: John Wiley & Sons, 1971.

King, I.M. *The Health Care System: Nursing Intervention Subsystem.* Werley, H. et al. Health Research: The Systems Approach. New York: Springer Publishing Co., 1976.

King, I.M. "How Does the Conceptual Framework Provide Structure for the Curriculum?" In *Curriculum Process for Developing or Revising BSN Programs.* New York: National League for Nursing, 1978.

King, I.M. Notes for Graduate Course in Curriculum and Instruction in Nursing, 1980.

King, I.M. *A Theory for Nursing: Systems, Concepts, Process.* New York: John Wiley & Sons, 1981.

King, I.M. National Survey of Philosophies of Nursing Education. *Western Journal of Nursing Research.* 6 (1984): 387–404.

Klausmeier, H.E.; Ghatala, E.S.; and Frayer, D.A. *Conceptual Learning and Development.* New York: Academic Press, 1974.

Kohl, H. *On Teaching.* New York: Schocken Books, 1976.

Kolb, Lawrence A. *Learning Style Inventory.* Boston: McBer and Company, 1978.

Krathwohl, D.R.; Bloom, B.S.; and Masia, B.B. *Taxonomy of Educational Objectives: Affective Domain.* New York: David McKay, 1964.

Kulik, J.A.; Kulik, Chen Lin; and Carmichael, K. "The Keller Plan in Science Teaching." *Science.* February 1, (1974): 379–83.

Lambertson, E. *Education for Nursing Leadership.* Philadelphia: J.B. Lippincott, 1958.

Lysaught, J. *An Abstract for Action.* New York: McGraw-Hill, 1970.

Maccia, E.S. "Theories of Instruction." In *Conceptual Models in Teacher Education,* edited by John R. Verduin, Jr. Washington, D.C.: AACTE, 1967.

McClellan, James E. *Philosophy of Education.* Englewood Cliffs, N.J.: Prentice-Hall, 1976.

Mager, Robert F. *Preparing Instructional Objectives.* Belmont, Ca.: Fearon Publishers, 1962.

Montag, M. *Education of Nurse Technicians.* New York: G.P. Putnam's Sons, 1951.

Montag, M. Education of Nurse Technicians. New York: G.P. Putnam's Sons, 1951.

Mueller, D.J. "Mastery Learning." *Teachers College Record.* 78 (1976):41–52.

National League for Nursing Education (NLNE). *A Curriculum Guide for Schools of Nursing.* New York: National League for Nursing Education, 1937.

National League for Nursing Education. *Standard Curriculum for Schools of Nursing.* Baltimore, Md.: Waverly Press, 1917.

National League for Nursing Education. *A Curriculum for Schools of Nursing.* New York: National League for Nursing Education, 1927.

Nelson, Sr. J. "The Thoughts of Martin Buber and Gabriel Marcel: Implications for Existentialism Encounters in Nursing." Unpublished doctoral dissertation. New York: Teachers' College, Columbia University, 1977.

Norman, E.M., and Haumann, L. "A Model for Judging Teacher Effectiveness." *Nurse Educator* III, 2, (1978):29–35.

Nunney, D.N., and Hill, J.E. "Personalized Educational Programs." *Audiovisual Instruction.* 17, 2 (1972):10–15.

Ozimek, Dorothy. *Relating the Open Curriculum to Accountability in Baccalaureate Education.* New York: National League for Nursing, 1976.

Parker, J. Cecil, and Rubin, Louis J. *Process as Content: Curricu-*

*lum Design and the Application of Knowledge.* Chicago: Rand McNally, 1966.

Patterson, J. and Zderad, L. *Humanistic Nursing.* New York: John Wiley & Sons, 1976.

Pfeiffer, John. *New Look at Education.* New York: Odyssey Press, 1968.

Phenix, Philip H. *Philosophies of Education.* New York: John Wiley & Sons, 1961.

Piaget, Jean. *The Conceptualization of Actions.* Chicago, Ill.: Chicago Institute for Psychoanalysis and Erikson Institute for Early Education, 1974.

Popham, W. James. *Criterion-Referenced Instruction.* Belmont, Ca.: Fearon Publishers, 1973.

Power, Edward J. *Philosophy of Education.* Englewood Cliffs, N.J.: Prentice-Hall, 1982.

Rogers, Carl R., and Coulson, N.R. *Freedom to Learn.* Columbus, Oh.: E. Merrill, 1969.

Simon, Herbert A. *Administrative Behavior.* New York: Macmillan, 1959.

Simpson, Elizabeth J. *The Classification of Educational Objectives: Psychomotor Domain.* Urbana, Ill.: University of Illinois Press, 1966.

Singer, R.N. *Psychomotor Domain: Movement Behavior.* Philadelphia: Lea and Febiger, 1972.

Stafford, L., and Graves, C.C. "Some Problems in Evaluating Teaching Effectiveness." *Nursing Outlook.* 26, 8 (1978): 494–97.

Steele, Shirley, *Educational Evaluation in Nursing.* New York: Charles B. Slack, 1978.

Steinaker, N.W., and Bell, M.R. *The Experiential Taxonomy: A New Approach to Teaching and Learning.* New York: Academic Press, 1979.

Stufflebeam, Daniel, et al. *Educational Evaluation and Decision Making.* Bloomington, Ind.: Phi Delta Kappa, 1971.

Suchman, J. "Inquiry Training." In *Conceptual Models in Teacher Education,* edited by John Verduin, Washington, D.C.: AACTE, 1967.

Taba, H. "Teaching Strategies for Cognitive Growth." In Verduin, J.R. *Conceptual Models in Teacher Education.* Washington, D.C.: AACTE (1967):16–26.

Tanner, Daniel, and Tanner, Laurel W. *Curriculum Development.* New York: Macmillan, 1980.

Taylor, E. "Of what is the nature of nursing?" *American Journal of Nursing.* 34, 5 (1934):473–476.

Torres, G., and Yura, H. *Today's Conceptual Framework: Its Relationship to the Curriculum Development Process.* New York: National League for Nursing, 1974.

Torres, G., and Stanton, M. *Curriculum Process in Nursing.* Englewood Cliffs, N.J.: Prentice-Hall, 1982.

Treece, E. "Philosophical Basis for Nursing Education." *International Nurses Review.* 21 (1974):13–15.

Tribbles, L. "Theories of Adult Education: Implications for Development of a Philosophy of Continuing Education in Nursing." *Journal of Continuing Education for Nursing.* 8(1977):25–28.

Tyler, Ralph N. *Basic Principles of Curriculum and Instruction.* Chicago: University of Chicago Press, 1949.

Ulsafer, J. "A Relationship of Existential Philosophy to Psychiatric Nursing." *Perspectives in Psychiatric Nursing.* 1(1976): 23–28.

Vaillot, Sr. C. *Commitment to Nursing.* Philadelphia: J.B. Lippincott, 1962.

Waltz, C.F.; Strickland, O.L.; and Lenz, E.R. *Measurement in Nursing Research.* Philadelphia: F.A. Davis, 1984.

Webb, Eugene J.; Campbell, Donald T.; Schwartz, Richard D.; and Sechrest, Lee. *Unobtrusive Measures: Nonreactive Research in the Social Sciences.* Chicago: Rand McNally, 1966.

Weil, Marsha, and Joyce, Bruce. *Information Processing Models of Teaching.* Englewood Cliffs, N.J.: Prentice-Hall, 1978.

Wiener, Norbert. *The Human Use of Human Beings.* New York: Avon, 1967.

Woodruff, Asahel D. *Basic Concepts of Teaching.* San Francisco: Chandler Publishing Company, 1961.

Yura, H. and Walsh, M. *The Nursing Process.* New York: Appleton-Century-Crofts, 1983.

Zasowska, Sr. A.A. "The Philosophy Index of Health Care Delivery in Our Culture." In *Health Care Dimensions.* M. Leninger, ed., Philadelphia: F.A. Davis, 1974, 1–16.

# A Rationale for Curriculum Development

## INTRODUCTION

The educational system in America has been allocated the responsibility for providing programs to help individuals learn skills for occupations and to learn concepts, skills, and values to become professionals. Teachers are expected to help individuals learn about self, about others, about being a citizen, about preserving the values of society, and about ways of coping with an increasing technological society.

Higher education is conceived to be a formal program of study in a community college, a senior college or a university leading to a specific degree. The purpose of Part II is to demonstrate the use of theoretical knowledge of learning, teaching, and curriculum presented in Part I to develop curricula for nursing in higher education. A rationale for developing a curriculum is discussed in Chapter 4. An undergraduate program with a major in nursing leading to a baccalaureate degree in nursing in a senior college or university is presented in Chapter 5. A curriculum leading to an associate degree in nursing in a community college is discussed in Chapter 6. Several factors to be considered in planning for articulation between associate degree and baccalaureate degree programs in nursing are identified in Chapter 7. Application of curriculum concepts to revision of ongoing programs is demonstrated in Chapter 8.

The complexity of knowledge and skills essential for professional nurses to function in health-care systems in the United States requires the development of educational programs to help students gain the knowledge and skills as efficiently and effectively as possible. A systems approach is one way to plan, implement, and evaluate the effectiveness of future-oriented curricula.

Every system has one or more goals. Generally, the purpose of an educational system is to prepare individuals to be useful, productive, and relatively happy citizens. Specifically, many educational programs prepare individuals for a variety of occupations and professions. In this chapter questions are asked and, when answered by faculty, provide information for decision making about curriculum and instruction.

Teachers help students acquire the values of the nursing profession through modeling behaviors, such as active participation in organized nursing, decision making for the profession, ability to identify and solve problems in nursing, and participation in, conducting, and utilizing research. An attitude toward lifelong learning is one of the values that can be portrayed by teachers. Teachers who demonstrate use of knowledge in nursing in health-care systems, who have visibility in health-care system as care givers and teachers, and who demonstrate collaborative relationships with health professionals, exhibit values in their behavior. Each individual learner brings some differences in knowledge, skills, interests, attitudes, and goals to an instructional situation. Diagnostic testing by teachers provides assessment data about these differences. Information from these assessments is helpful for teachers to plan learning activities and instructional strategies, and to use resources to meet the goals of learners.

If teachers in nursing education programs expect students to gain the knowledge and skills required to function as professional nurses and technical nurses at the completion of a program, strategies for mastery learning will ensure equality of learning outcomes for students enrolled in the programs. Mastery learning has provided a rationale for the development of competency-based curricula. Several programs, including external degree programs, have implemented competency-based curricula. A basic assumption about teaching for mastery learning is that teachers must select strategies that consider individual differences in learners and provide learning activities to promote student learning. Answering specific questions will provide information for faculty groups prior to making decisions about the kind of curriculum they will develop.

## INFORMATION FOR DECISION MAKING

Faculty members in nursing in higher education have diverse backgrounds in nursing, education, and research. Each individual faculty member brings to the group differences in perceptions about curriculum and instruction. These individual differences are recognized but at the same time need a focus for group deliberations. A series of questions is presented as a basis for thinking about a rationale for a nursing education curriculum. As faculty members answer these questions, similarities and differences in philosophy and knowledge emerge, and the group begins to learn how to identify areas of common agreement. Questions are presented and examples of answers are given. After faculty members respond to these questions, a curriculum can be developed.

### 1. To whom are professional nurses responsible and accountable?

When society decides that a group of individuals are professionals, these individuals, as an organized profession and as individuals, are responsible and accountable to the public for whom they provide an essential service. As a profession, the members are self-regulating, and so they promulgate a code of ethics and define and disseminate standards of care to be implemented (ANA, 1976; ANA, 1978). Professionals also evaluate the effectiveness of the care given through the quality assurance programs implemented in health-care agencies.

### 2. What is the relationship of nursing to other professions?

In most health-care agencies, nurses are the coordinators of care. Professional nurses recognize an interdependent role and also exert leadership in establishing collaborative relationships with other health-care professionals in the systems. "Nurses are partners with physicians, social workers and allied health professionals in promoting health, in preventing disease, and in managing patient care" (King, 1976, p. 52). The professional nurse is represented on an interdisciplinary health team and in some situations is the leader of the team because of the information gathered by nurses that identifies and sometimes helps solve client problems. The professional nurse on the health team is the synthesizer of information and shares observations, measurements, and inferences with other members of the health team.

### 3. What is the relationship of nursing to the health-care system?

Professional nurses, as employees of health-care systems, have a legal relationship called master–servant. At the same time, nurses are licensed to practice as professionals in certain states, and the law governing their licenses defines that practice. The relationship at best has a built-in potential conflict that must be clarified in the process of educating a professional nurse.

### 4. What is the relationship of professional nursing to the community, the nation, and the world?

As members of a profession, nurses are expected to become members of their professional organization, the American Nurses Association. As members of this organization, nurses are members of the International Council of Nurses, which holds quadrennial meetings in different countries. Also, nurses are members of their state nurses associations. Under the recently revised structure of the American Nurses Association (1982), state nurses associations are the constituent members of the organization.

As citizens, nurses are members of a democratic society in which the national government is elected by the people. Elected officials represent us in making decisions to protect our rights and our freedom, and to preserve our society. Nurses are also active citizens participating in the political process at local, state, and national levels of government.

### 5. Where do professional nurses perform their functions?

Nurses serve in many roles in a variety of social organizations of different sizes and structures, and with a variety of persons. Some of these organizations are schools, industries, and official and voluntary health agencies. In addition, over 50 percent of employed nurses perform functions in hospitals of different sizes, controls, and purposes. No other group of health professionals provides services in such a variety of social organizations. Nurses perform functions in families, in neighborhood clinics, in clinics for the elderly, in health assessment and health education in private practice, and in other roles.

In hospitals, nurses function as staff nurses, head nurses, supervisors, assistant and associate directors, directors and vice-presidents for nursing. In these roles, they are practitioners, teachers, managers, administrators, and consultants. A primary purpose of hospitals is service for the sick, but nurses also function as researchers and teachers.

The expansion of nursing homes and health care for the elderly has increased the demand for nurses to direct and supervise care for the aging in our population. Nurses function in local health agencies, in the state department of health, and in federal health services. "Occupational health nurses have been employed for many years by business and industry to provide health care for adult workers" (King, 1971, pp. 55–58).

### 6. Who decides the functions of professional nurses?

Society identifies the need for social services; however, the individuals who are members of professions determine the role and functions to be performed. The professionals also determine the educational requirements for that service. An organized profession promulgates a code of ethics which indicates social responsibility. In order to protect the public, laws are passed in each state that provide legal boundaries for professional functions.

### 7. What are the goals of professional nursing education?

An overall goal for professional nursing education is to prepare individuals who will be intelligent citizens and will use their knowledge as a basis for understanding human behavior. Graduates will use the knowledge and skills of the profession and incorporate its values to deliver effective nursing care in a variety of community health-care settings. Each educational program states specific goals for its graduates. The major goal is to provide qualified individuals to practice nursing as either professional or as technical nurses. Since nursing is licensed in each state, one goal is to pass the state licensing examination to legally practice nursing.

When a faculty group has discussed nursing in relation to society, to other health professionals, and to the profession, more specific questions should be addressed that relate to the educational systems and elements in the curriculum in specific educational programs. A series of questions with examples of responses are presented.


## WHAT IS HIGHER EDUCATION?


Higher education has been traditionally defined as formal educational programs organized within post-secondary institutions chartered by the state to offer programs leading to specific degrees. More recently, innovations in education have been reported whereby nontraditional educational programs have been offered leading to degrees. These are called external degree programs (Lenburg, 1976). For further information consult journals in nursing and in higher education.

The community college movement gathered momentum in the early 1960's to implement the philosophy that all citizens in this country should have equality of educational opportunity. Initially in the United States junior colleges were founded to offer the first two years of college before students transferred to senior colleges to complete their undergraduate studies. Today, community colleges have replaced junior colleges and have multiple purposes, one of which is to offer formal programs leading to preparation for an occupation. Another purpose is to provide educational and recreational opportunities for citizens in a community. A third is the original transfer purpose. Community colleges in most states are organized within the system of higher education.

## WHAT IS EDUCATION FOR THE PROFESSION OF NURSING?

Education for most professions is offered as formal programs in colleges and universities. The prerequisites for entrance into a professional curriculum vary with each profession and its educational standards. Whitehead (1948) distinguished between crafts in the ancient world and professions in the modern world. He explained that a craft is based on customary practices and changed by trial and error. On the other hand, a profession is based on activities that are subject to theoretical analysis and altered by conclusions derived from that analysis (pp. 73-74).

The professional nurse of today and tomorrow must be able to assess systematically clients' abilities to function in social roles, to identify alterations in normal functioning, to take action based on theoretical knowledge, and to conduct evaluations of actions to determine effectiveness of nursing care. Professional nurses will be expected to add to the body of knowledge through studies of practice and the use of research findings when appropriate. Professionals contribute to deliberations and goal setting by a health team to provide quality health care. Professionals implement the standards of nursing care of the profession and promulgate the code for nurses in ethical decision making. Professional nurses are expected to set mutual goals with clients and patients, to write nursing orders to be carried out by all nursing personnel according to their level of ability to function as members of the nursing team, and to write discharge notes that show the effectiveness of nursing care delivered.

The technical nurse of today and tomorrow will assist the professional nurse in carrying out the means identified to attain nursing goals established. The technical nurse will participate as an active member of the nursing team and demonstrate technical competencies in nursing situations. The technical nurse will increase knowledge and skills and assist in evaluating the nursing care given. In this age of high technology, many technical nurses will be essential in the delivery of skilled nursing care. Technical nurses will function primarily in secondary and tertiary care settings. Through continuing education they will increase their knowledge and competencies.

## SIMILARITIES AND DIFFERENCES BETWEEN PROFESSIONAL AND TECHNICAL NURSING

Generally, the graduates of a baccalaureate program have had four years in formal education and have been exposed to the major ideas of several fields of study that contribute to knowledge of society, individuals, and groups. The nursing major is designed so that students use knowledge and skills from other areas of study.

Generally, the graduates of an associate degree program have two years in formal education with an introductory course in a few fields of knowledge related to nursing. The nursing courses are designed to provide basic knowledge and skills in nursing so the graduates can begin to function under supervision in health-care agencies.

**Similarities in Both Programs.**   Graduates of both programs will have:

1. Knowledge of and commitment to accepted values based on ethical principles consistent with the nursing profession and a democratic society.

2. Knowledge of the fundamental social, political, and economic problems in society.

3. Consistency in their view of life, which encompasses basic human needs, and consistency in their social expression and relationship to others, to a higher being, and to society.

4. Knowledge of the role and functions of technical and professional nurses in society and the ability to func-

tion in a collaborative way to deliver effective and safe nursing care.

5. Basic knowledge and skills in secondary and tertiary care systems.

**Differences in Both Programs.** In the baccalaureate program, the number and kinds of courses in basic sciences, behavioral sciences, and the humanities provide the students with theoretical knowledge related to nursing. Critical thinking is required, and students increase intellectual skills in analysis and interpretation through the use of inductive and deductive reasoning. Students are expected to express themselves clearly in writing and verbally as well as to listen, to read with comprehension, and to understand messages in verbal and nonverbal communications. Students are introduced to theories in a number of fields of study and learn how to explore ideas, to challenge current ways of doing things, and to become familiar with the past as a way of understanding themselves and others in a changing world. Students learn the role of the manager in complex organizations, such as health care agencies. They gain experience in functioning as individuals and as members of groups within selected health-care organizations. Students are able to identify problems and to gather facts for making decisions and for making discriminative judgments based on scientific knowledge.

In associate degree programs, students gain the ability to think logically and to express themselves verbally and in writing. They begin to develop a concept of self as a basis for knowing others. Students learn the role and functions of technical nurses and gain the ability to function as members of the nursing team. Students have the ability to use basic skills in giving routine nursing care. Specifically, the differences are in the areas of communication, critical thinking, discriminative judgment, and decision making in complex nursing situations. Graduates of baccalaureate programs are able to assume the role of professional nurse after some orientation to the health-care system. Graduates of associate degree programs are able to assume the role of technical nurse after an orientation to the health-care system and with supervision of the professional nurse. Similarities and differences between baccalaureate and associate degree graduates are:

| TECHNICAL | PROFESSIONAL |
|---|---|
| Assessment of client status: | Assessment of client status: |
| Records and reports findings to professional nurse. | Uses reliable tools to collect, analyze, and interpret data. |
| Uses direct and indirect observation techniques to gather data. | Uses participant and nonparticipant observation techniques systematically to collect data, interpret data, and make a nursing diagnosis. |
| Assists professional nurses to implement means selected to achieve goals. | Identifies goals to be achieved *with* clients when they can participate in goal setting and *for* clients when they cannot participate in goal setting. |
| Carries out nursing orders. | Writes nursing orders that identify means to achieve goals. |
| Records process used to achieve goals. | |
| Participates in coordinating nursing care with nursing team. | Evaluates goal attainment. |
| | Coordinates nursing care with nursing and health team. |
| Applies research findings identified by professional nurses. | Uses research findings to verify observations, goals, and nursing orders. |
| Participates in evaluation of goals attained to determine effectiveness of care. | Determines effectiveness of care by evaluation of goals attained. |

**Functions of Professional Nurses.**  In the Nursing Practice Acts in some states, the law enumerates the functions of nursing. These functions are summarized as follows:

1.  Supervision and management of care, which requires the application of principles based on the biological, physical, and behavioral sciences and humanities.

2. Observation of behaviors in the form of reactions, symptoms of disease and illness, both mental and physical, that requires use of scientific knowledge from biological, physical, and behavioral sciences.

3. Accurate recording and reporting of facts about patients and clients and evaluation of the total situation.

4. Implementation of nursing goals through the application of appropriate techniques and procedures.

5. Direction of the nursing care of individuals and groups and providing for essential health education to help them maintain their health.

6. Supervision of nursing personnel.

7. Implementation of physician's orders for treatments and medications based on nurse's knowledge and understanding of same.

In addition to the above functions, professional nurses, through interactions with patients and clients, communicate information and mutually set goals to be attained whenever possible. The means that are available to achieve goals are explored and agreed on by nurses and patients. When patients cannot participate, nurses will set goals for them or consult with family members. All personnel work toward attainment of the patient's goals. The professional nurse evaluates the effectiveness of nursing when goals are attained. Implementation of a human process of interactions that lead to transactions between the nurse and patient will result in goal attainment. Both individuals learn in the process of these interactions and gain some satisfaction in achieving goals.

**Functions of the Technical Nurse.** Graduates of associate degree programs provide general nursing care with supervision from professional nurses. Technical nurses continue to develop their technical competencies in general nursing and, with continuing education, move to higher levels of technical nursing in specialized care areas. The technical nurse works with professional nurses and assists in planning, implementing, and evaluating the nursing care of individuals and groups.

**What is the Organizing Focus for a Curriculum?**   A conceptual framework identifies the structure for a curriculum. Concepts are the organizing elements in the framework and guide faculty in the identification of essential content for the curriculum. A conceptual framework is formulated after faculty members have developed at least a working philosophy of nursing education. Two essential components for writing a rationale for a curriculum are a stated philosophy of nursing education and a conceptual framework that is derived from the philosophy. Suggestions for writing a philosophy and formulating a conceptual framework were presented in Chapters 2 and 3. Faculty groups may select a conceptual framework published in nursing literature or they may develop their own framework for their specific program.

**What Knowledge is Essential for Nurses to Provide Professional Nursing Care?**   Nurses must have knowledge about human beings and human behavior in a variety of situations. This knowledge is derived from basic and behavior sciences and the humanities. Recently, nurses have constructed theories and conceptual models from which theories can be derived. The scientific movement to continue to identify a body of knowledge essential for professional nursing has reached adulthood. Hypotheses are being generated from these models and theories are tested in research to describe, explain, and predict events and actions in nursing situations.

**What Skills are Essential for Nurses to Function in the Professional Role?**   Several basic skills are essential for nurses to function in their role. Observation is an example of a skill, along with measurement of parameters of human beings, situations, and external environment. These two skills are basic because through the information gathered from the use of skills, nurses make inferences, judgments, and decisions for actions to help individuals promote, regain, and maintain health.

Communication is another skill required in every nursing situation. (See King, 1981, pp. 62–80 for references). Interviews and questionnaires are techniques for gathering observation data. Increased technology in health care systems has demanded that nurses have knowledge of physics in understanding machines that are used particularly in critical care areas. Some of the skills required to understand and work with machines may be considered advanced technical skills in specialized areas of practice. Health assessment skills, introduced as basic skills in a curriculum, are recent additions to the nurse's repertoire. Many resources are available for information about these skills.

**What are the Values of Organized Nursing?** A quotation from the Code for Nurses (ANA, 1976) gives some idea of values of nursing.

> The Code for Nurses is based on belief about the nature of individuals, nursing, health and society. Recipients and providers of nursing services are viewed as individuals and groups who possess basic rights and responsibilities, and whose values and circumstances command respect at all times. Nursing encompasses the promotion and restoration of health, the prevention of illness, and the alleviation of suffering (p. 2).

A code demonstrates a profession's commitment, accountability, and responsibility to clients for a service deemed essential by society. "The requirements of the Code may exceed but are never less than those of the law" (ANA, 1976, p. 1).

Values of the profession are expressed in the published *Standards of Nursing Practice* (ANA, 1973). Standards provide a measure to judge the competence of the members of a profession (King, 1981, pp. 12–13).

Following faculty members' deliberations about the philosophy, conceptual framework, and responses to the questions presented in this chapter, small groups may begin to write program objectives or competencies expected of students at graduation. Some of the ideas presented are used in subsequent chapters to present hypothetical curricula for professional and technical nursing programs.

# chapter
# 5

# A Curriculum Leading to a Baccalaureate Degree

The overall aim of an undergraduate program with a major in nursing is guidance of individuals through planned learning activities to achieve the specific knowledge, skills, values, and attitudes characteristic of professional nurses. Upon completion of the program, graduates are able to practice professional nursing in any setting after orientation to the work situation.

Characteristics of graduates of baccalaureate programs in nursing have been identified by faculty and administrators in baccalaureate programs. The following characteristics were approved by the professional membership of the Council of Baccalaureate and Higher Degree Programs of the National League for Nursing Education:

Utilize theory in making decisions on nursing practice.

Use nursing practice as a means of gathering data for refining and extending that practice.

Synthesize theoretical and empirical knowledge from the physical and behavioral sciences and humanities with nursing theory and practice.

Assess health status and health potential; plan, implement, and evaluate nursing care of individuals, families, and communities.

Improve service to the client by continually evaluating the effectiveness of nursing intervention and revising it accordingly.

Accept individual responsibility and accountability for the choice of nursing intervention and its outcome.

Evaluate research for the applicability of its findings to nursing actions.

Utilize leadership skills through involvement with others in meeting health needs and nursing goals.

Collaborate with colleagues and citizens on the interdisciplinary health team to promote the health and welfare of people.

Participate in identifying and effecting needed change to improve delivery within specific health care systems.

Participate in identifying community and societal health needs and in designing nursing roles to meet these needs (NLN, 1978).

Nursing is a profession sanctioned by society because it provides a social service to meet a social need. The focus of nursing is on the human being, a dynamic individual, whose perceptions influence behavior and health.

Elements shown in Figure 5.1 will be discussed to demonstrate a process for developing a curriculum for an undergraduate program with a major in nursing leading to a baccalaureate degree. The first element states a philosophy of nursing education from which the second element, a conceptual framework, is identified. After a faculty group states a philosophy and designs a framework, objectives are formulated. When the faculty has reached agreement on these three elements, courses can be identified. Faculty select courses in other fields of study that provide prerequisite knowledge for entrance into the nursing major. Following these decisions, the nursing courses can be designed. A hypothetical curriculum is proposed to demonstrate the use of ideas in previous chapters. Any resemblance to current programs is purely coincidental.

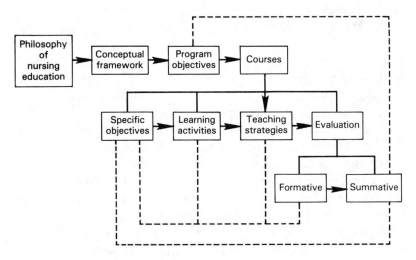

**Figure 5.1**
Curriculum and Instruction Process

## A HYPOTHETICAL BACCALAUREATE PROGRAM

Philosophical assumptions about teaching, learning, curriculum, and the discipline of nursing form the basis for decision making about the kind of curriculum developed in higher education. These assumptions are made explicit and serve to guide the development of a curriculum and the instructional design.

The overall purpose of this hypothetical program is the education of individuals to function after graduation in the role of professional nurses. The philosophy and conceptual framework provide the organizing elements for the curriculum.

### Philosophy of Nursing Education

The statement of philosophy for a curriculum in a hypothetical College of Nursing is in keeping with the purposes of the University, a democratic society, and the aims of professional nursing. The philosophy is based on assumptions about human beings, society, health-care systems, health, higher education, learning, teaching, nursing, and nursing education.

Human beings are open systems in continuous transactions with the environment. Human beings are unique individuals of intrinsic worth who are capable of relating, communicating, thinking, choosing, and making decisions on the basis of their perceptions, background experiences, interests, and goals. Individuals function in an environment of social systems in a society. Human beings have a right to health care. They have also a responsibility to engage in health practices.

American society offers citizens the right to freedom, justice, and protection under the Constitution. A variety of social systems has been organized to help individuals achieve goals. Examples of these systems are: the family, educational systems, work systems, recreational systems, religious and community organizations, and health-care systems. The social systems are conceived to be the environments within which individuals grow and develop. Local, state, and federal governments provide for health-care systems through public and private sources.

Health-care delivery systems have been categorized into primary, secondary, and tertiary care. Ethical and legal issues have been identified that relate to health care of individuals and groups and to the high technology used for treatment and therapy. Society gives the responsibility for preserving the dignity of human beings in treatment and care to health professionals to help individuals maintain a state of health in which they can function in their social roles.

Health relates to the way individuals cope with the stressors of growth and development while the individuals are functioning in the culture in which they were born and to which they attempt to conform (King, 1971, p. 67). Health is defined as "dynamic life experiences of a human being, which implies continuous adjustment to stressors in the internal and external environment through optimum use of one's resources to achieve maximum potential for daily living" (King, 1981, p. 5). Initial health practices are learned within the family.

The goals of nursing include health promotion, health maintenance and restoration, care of the ill, and care of individuals who are dying (King, 1981, p. 4). Nursing is a process of action, reaction, interaction, and transaction whereby nurse and client share information about their perceptions in a nursing situation. Through purposeful communication they identify specific goals, problems, or concerns. They explore means to achieve a goal and agree to the means to use to reach a goal. When clients participate in goal setting, they interact with nurses to move toward goal attainment in most situations (King, 1981, p. 2). When individuals cannot actively participate, nurses set goals for clients and with families of clients. Professional nursing involves the use of knowledge and the nurse's use of self in assessing, planning, diagnosing, setting goals, implementing, and evaluating nursing care to meet the needs of individuals and groups. Through their actions, professional nurses demonstrate responsibility and accountability to society. Nurses function independently as professionals and collaboratively with health professionals to meet the health-care needs of people.

Learning is self-activity and requires involvement of individuals in the process. Learning is characterized by thinking and decision making. Learning is an individual experience as each person grows and develops. Each individual has a personal learning style and individual goals and learns at a different rate of speed. Feedback and reinforcement facilitate learning.

Teaching is a complex process characterized by planning, selecting, assessing, organizing, sequencing, facilitating, guiding, implementing, and evaluating individual learners and programs to achieve goals. A climate is provided for teachers to have the freedom to teach and students to have the freedom to learn. Teaching is goal directed and based on learner's needs, interests, and goals.

Education for professional nursing aims to prepare individuals who are active participants in planned learning activities in a formal educational system. Through these activities, individuals learn a scientific way of thinking about nursing and about health care. They gain the specific knowledge, skills, and values essential to practice as professional nurses. In addition, individuals make decisions based on relevant information and act consistently and reasonably as members of a profession and a democratic society.

The philosophical assumptions serve to guide a faculty group to formulate a framework for the curriculum. The conceptual framework for this College of Nursing follows the theme in this book, which is to use a systems approach to curriculum and instruction.

## CONCEPTUAL FRAMEWORK FOR THE CURRICULUM

A general systems framework is proposed to provide structure for the curriculum. The three dynamic interacting systems are shown in Figure 5.2. Personal systems in the diagram relate to each individual. Interpersonal systems are described as dyads (two individuals interacting); triads (three individuals interacting; or small and large groups of four or more individuals interacting). Social systems are described as those groups that form to achieve specific purposes within a society, such as family,

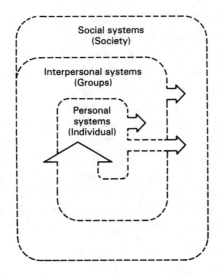

**Figure 5.2**
Dynamic Interacting Systems (From: I.M.
King, *A Theory for Nursing: Concepts, Process,
and Systems*. New York: John Wiley, 1981,
p. 11.)

school, business and industry, churches, hospitals, and other
health-care organizations. Social systems provide the environment within which individuals and groups develop, grow, learn,
and perform their functions in life.

Every system has goals. The goal for nursing is health
(King, 1971). This goal includes health promotion, health maintenance, and prevention of disease, illness, and disability. In
addition, the goal includes care for individuals with illness, disease, and disability, to help them achieve a functional state of
health, and to assist individuals to die with dignity. The focus
for nursing is helping individuals who make up groups, such as
families, to maintain their health, and providing assistance to
those with functional disabilities to learn how to cope with
them.

Major concepts are selected within each of the three dynamic interacting systems. A major concept that gives us knowledge
about self, about others, and about environment is perception.

Concepts related to perception are self, body image, learning, growth, development, time, and space.

A major concept that gives us knowledge about interpersonal systems is human interaction. Concepts related to interaction are communication, transaction, role, and stress.

A major concept that gives us knowledge about social systems is organization. Concepts related to organization are power, control, authority, status, role, and decision making.

This framework with relevant concepts identified in each of the three dynamic interacting systems provides the organizing elements for the curriculum proposed for educating individuals to become professional nurses. From a stated philosophy and this conceptual framework, program objectives are formulated.

### Program Objectives

Individuals who select a program of study in a university should know the outcomes expected of them at the completion of the program. Several factors determine the type of objectives to be achieved to become a professional nurse. Educational standards for entrance into professional nursing are influenced by professional standards of practice. Another factor is the code of ethics for the profession. Other factors are influenced by the need for professional nursing services in society and the complex and varied health care delivery systems. The following objectives are suggested for a curriculum to prepare professional nurses.

At the completion of the program, graduates will:

1. Integrate knowledge of human–environment interactions to promote health, maintain health, regain health, and prevent illness in planning, implementing, and evaluating nursing care of individuals and groups.

2. Interpret the interrelationship of perceptions, communications, and transactions in human interactions of nurses, clients, families, and health professionals in helping individuals who are ill return to health.

3. Integrate ethical values of professional nursing in decision making in nursing and health care.

4. Use relevant knowledge from basic sciences, behavioral sciences, the humanities, and nursing in planning, implementing, and evaluating effectiveness of nursing care for individuals and groups in primary, secondary, and tertiary health-care systems.

5. Demonstrate responsibility and accountability for nursing care of individuals and groups.

6. Interpret the independent and collaborative functions of professional nurses.

7. Use a theory of goal attainment for nursing in working with individuals and groups to facilitate the optimum health needed to function in social roles.

8. Demonstrate mastery in performance of basic and advanced technical skills.

9. Formulate a life plan for continuing personal and professional development.

Before proceeding to identify courses for the curriculum, faculty groups should look at the *balance* in the program objectives. A brief review shows that objective 8 relates to technical skills in nursing, and represents the psychomotor domain of knowledge. Knowledge is essential in the practice of professional nursing, and objectives 1, 2, 3, and 6 in the cognitive domain are suggested. Objectives, 4, 5, 7, and 9 in the affective domain are presented. The importance of the interrelationship between the cognitive and affective domains of knowledge is reflected in the objectives and shows balance. Objectives of this type provide the road map for faculty groups to design a program of study.

From overall program objectives, which are more general in nature than course objectives, courses are planned by faculty. The program objectives guide faculty both in the selection of courses that provide knowledge prerequisite for nursing courses and in the organization of courses for nursing.

**Prerequisite Courses.** When decisions have been made about philosophy, conceptual framework, and program objectives, faculty members determine prerequisite courses for the nursing major. Based on ideas in the stated philosophy and conceptual framework, a variety of courses are recommended from the major disciplines.

Behavioral sciences include introductory courses in sociology, psychology, anthropology, political science, and economics. Courses from the biophysical sciences would include physics, biology, anatomy, physiology, biochemistry, microbiology, and immunology. Courses in the humanities are English, which includes communications, art and music appreciation, logic, philosophy, and history. Courses selected from various disciplines provide knowledge prerequisite for entering the nursing major and for a liberal education.

**Courses in the Major.** Nursing courses build on knowledge obtained from the basic sciences, behavioral sciences, and the humanities. Courses and credit hours for the nursing major are:

| TITLES | CREDIT HOURS |
|---|---|
| Historical and Philosophical Foundations of Nursing | 3 |
| Theories of Nursing | 3 |
| Ethical and Legal Dimensions of Nursing | 3 |
| Principles of Teaching and Learning in Client Education | 3 |
| Introduction to Nursing: Concepts, Process, and Skills | 3 |
| Practicum in Introduction to Nursing | 3 |
| Basis Skills Laboratory | 2 |
| Nursing in the Community | 3 |
| Practicum in Community Nursing | 3 |
| Nursing in Groups | 3 |
| Practicum in Nursing in Groups | 3 |
| Nursing of Individuals | 9 |

| | |
|---|---|
| Practicum in Nursing of Individuals | 9 |
| Role and Functions of a Professional Nurse | 2 |
| Practicum in Role and Functions of a Professional Nurse | 4 |
| Electives in nursing and other disciplines | 6-12 |

Sixty-six credit hours are designed for meeting the requirements for a nursing major. This total includes six to twelve credit hours of electives.

Attention is given to *sequence* when faculty groups select courses and plan for instruction. Sequence means that teachers believe that prior knowledge and skills are essential before learners can move on to new activities and advanced skills. Piaget's studies of the intellectual development of children, Bruner's ideas about the structure of subject matter in a curriculum, and Bloom and colleagues' work at the University of Chicago, support Tyler's idea of sequence as a major component in organizing a curriculum.

**Placement of Courses in the Nursing Major.** The placement of courses in the junior and senior years of the educational program reflect faculty beliefs about the sequence of learning experiences. When the university operates on a trimester basis, course placement is suggested as follows:

| JUNIOR YEAR | CREDIT HOURS |
|---|---|
| *First Semester* | |
| Historical and Philosophical Foundations of Nursing | 3 |
| Theories of Nursing | 3 |
| Introduction to Nursing: Concepts, Process, and Skills | 3 |
| Practicum—Introduction to Nursing | 3 |
| Elective | 3 |
| *Second Semester* | |
| Principles of Teaching and Learning in Client Education | 3 |
| Nursing in the Community | 3 |
| Practicum in Community Nursing | 3 |

| | |
|---|---|
| Ethical and Legal Dimensions of Nursing | 3 |
| Elective | 3 |
| *Third Semester* | |
| Nursing in Groups | 3 |
| Practicum in Nursing in Groups | 3 |
| **SENIOR YEAR** | **CREDIT HOURS** |
| *First Semester* | |
| Nursing of Individuals | 6 |
| Practicum in Nursing of Individuals | 6 |
| Elective | 3 |
| *Second Semester* | |
| Nursing of Individuals | 3 |
| Practicum in Nursing of Individuals | 3 |
| Role and Functions of a Professional Nurse | 6 |
| Elective | 3 |

None of the above courses are developed in detail in this book; however, examples are given to demonstrate the use of a conceptual approach to curriculum and instruction. When faculty members have made decisions about the nursing courses to be taught and the sequence in which learners will enroll in the courses, a format for instructional planning, shown in Figure 5.3, is useful.

The process begins first with a formulation of objectives for each course in terms of behavior outcomes in the cognitive, affective, and psychomotor domains. Second, selection of learning activities are made so students can practice the behaviors they are expected to achieve. Third, teaching strategies are selected that will provide guidance, feedback, and reinforcement for learners. Fourth, learning materials related to objectives are prepared. Fifth, formative evaluation is a process of feedback for corrective action by learners, if necessary. This process is an ongoing teacher function to facilitate learning during the learning process. Summative evaluation is planned and time established for the teacher to evaluate the learner's achievement of the objectives. This evaluation is used for grading in a system that requires a grade at the completion of a module or a course.

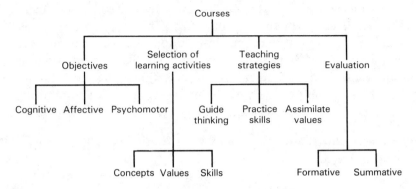

**Figure 5.3**

Instructional Process

For purposes of illustration, one course in this hypothetical curriculum will be developed. Two modules in the course are developed in detail to demonstrate the relation of the instructional process outlined in Figure 5.3 to program objectives, conceptual framework, and philosophy.

A format is used to show one approach for preparing course materials. The number and title of the course is given. This is followed with a course description. Course objectives are written in behavioral terms and categorized under the cognitive, affective, and psychomotor domains of knowledge. This categorization assists faculty in checking for balance in the course. This approach guides faculty to select appropriate and specific learning experiences so students can practice the behaviors expected in achieving course objectives.

The examples given in the two modules for writing objectives are traditional. However, at the end of the first module, two examples are given for those faculty who are or will be developing performance objectives related to mastery learning. This type of objective was proposed by Mager (1962) and includes the who, what, how, and where approach.

Following the statement of course objectives, the modules are identified and developed. Teachers include selected readings and a relevant bibliography for each course.

**Course Title:** Introduction to Nursing

**Course Description:**   A general systems framework for nursing is emphasized in which concepts of perception, self, body image, communication, interactions, transactions, health, environment, and activities of daily living are developed. Skills in observation, communication, interactions, transactions, history taking, health assessment of individuals, and assessment of a community and health practices are acquired.

**Course Objectives:**   At the completion of this course, a student will be able to:

1. Discuss a general systems framework for nursing and a theory of goal attainment.

2. Verify accuracy of his or her perception of patient/ client status with patient/client perception of health status.

3. Demonstrate communication, both verbal and non-verbal, in gathering reliable information through participant and nonparticipant observations of individuals of all age groups.

4. Identify at least five common psychosocial variables in nurse–patient and nurse–family interactions.

5. Identify the dependency of a patient/client from each age group in performing activities of daily living.

6. Demonstrate skill in health assessment of individuals in each of the age groups.

7. Describe similarities and differences in health-care agencies in which nurses function.

The course objectives were planned to introduce students to the framework of the curriculum and its relationship to a nursing theory of goal attainment.

An approach to crosscheck the way course objectives help learners achieve program objectives is shown in Figure 5.4. The course objectives and the module objectives are written to pro-

COURSE OBJECTIVES

| PROGRAM OBJECTIVES | N.R. 301 INTRO-DUCTION TO NR | N.R. 302 PRACTICUM |
|---|---|---|
| Integrate knowledge of human environment interactions to promote health, maintain health, regain health and prevent illness in planning, implementing and evaluating nursing care of individuals and groups. | X | X |
| Interpret interrelationship of perceptions, communications, transactions in human interactions of nurses, clients, families, and health professionals in helping individuals who are ill return to health. | X | X |
| Integrate ethical values of professional nursing in decision making in nursing and health care. | | |
| Use relevant knowledge from basic sciences, behavioral sciences, humanities and nursing in planning, implementing and evaluating effectiveness of nursing care for individuals and groups in primary, secondary and tertiary health care systems. | X | X |
| Demonstrate responsibility and accountability for nursing care of individuals and groups. | X | X |
| Interpret the independent and collaborative functions of professional nurses. | X | X |
| Use a theory of goal attainment for nursing in working with individuals and groups to facilitate optimum health to function in usual social roles | | |
| Demonstrate mastery in performance of basic and advanced technical skills. | X | X |
| Formulate a life plan for continuing personal and professional development. | | |

**Figure 5.4**

Relationship of Course Objectives to Program Objectives

vide specific opportunities in the cognitive, affective, and psychomotor domains of learning. For example, in the course proposed here, objectives 1, 5, and 7 are cognitive; objectives 2 and 4 are affective; and objectives 3 and 6 are psychomotor. The objectives are written to show relationships which facilitate faculty members' choice of learning activities. From course objectives, the objectives of each module are written to help students achieve the course objectives. Figure 5.5 presents an example of crosschecking to show the relationship between module and course objectives. For the first course in the nursing major in a hypothetical curriculum the modules are identified as follows:

Module 1. General systems framework and introduction to observation and measurement skills.

Module 2. Health as a goal: A nursing theory of goal attainment.

Module 3. Personal systems are individuals and interpersonal systems are groups.

Module 4. Assessment skills of observations and measurements.

Module 5. Concepts of perception, learning, self, and body image.

Module 6. Concepts of communication, transaction, and interaction.

Module 7. Social systems as environment.

Module 8. Role and functions of professional nurses in health-care agencies.

The first module introduces students to the course, teachers' expectations of learners, and learners' expectations of teachers. Each module is organized to let the students know the overall course and then to learn concepts, process, and skills as a basis for requirements in subsequent courses that help them achieve a goal of becoming a professional nurse.

| NR 301 Introduction to Nursing Course Objectives | \multicolumn{8}{c}{Module Objectives} |
|---|---|

| NR 301 Introduction to Nursing Course Objectives | 1 | 2 | 3 | 4 | 5 | 6 | 7 | 8 |
|---|---|---|---|---|---|---|---|---|
| Discuss a general systems framework and theory of goal attainment for nursing. | X | X | X | X | X | X | X | X |
| Verify accuracy of one's perception of client/patient with client/patient perception of his/her health status. | | X | X | X | X | X | | X |
| Demonstrate communication, both verbal and nonverbal, in gathering reliability information through participant and nonparticipant observations of individuals of all age levels. | | X | X | X | X | X | X | X |
| Identify at least five common psychosocial variables in nurse-patient and nurse-family interactions | | X | X | | X | X | X | X |
| Identify the dependency of a patient/client from each age group in performing activities of daily living. | | X | | X | X | X | X | X |
| Demonstrate skill in health assessment of individuals at each of the age levels. | | X | | X | | X | X | X |
| Describe similarities and differences in health care agencies in which nurses perform their functions. | | X | X | | | | X | X |

**Figure 5.5**

Relationship between Course Objectives and Module Objectives

The first two modules are developed in detail and the same format is used to develop the remaining modules. The ideas presented in the firsᴛ two modules are an approach to demonstrate a conceptually-based course in a nursing curriculum. The process for developing concepts can be found in several sources (King, 1975, 1981). Students are provided with a selected bibliography so they can begin to read relevant literature. Students are expected to read studies and articles about each concept. From the readings, they synthesize information for themselves. From the literature review, students identify characteristics of each concept and derive a working definition for themselves. Throughout the program they continue to develop their knowledge of each concept in the outlines. This process for developing concepts gives learners substantive knowledge that is retained for use at a later time. Since the nursing major in this hypothetical curriculum is based on a nursing conceptual framework (King, 1971, 1981), the major concepts are developed as substantive knowledge that is essential for becoming a professional nurse The students are introduced to the overall framework in the first module in the first course so they have a picture of the total curriculum. This is based on a belief about learning that one moves from the whole to specific elements and back to the whole in the learning process of developing one's knowledge and skills in a field of study.

For the reader who perceives this approach of whole–part–whole in learning as antithetical to a person-centered philosophy with emphasis on the unity of the learner or on wholism, the following quote should help change that perception:

> A philosophy that sets high store on the unity of the person is altogether praiseworthy; but it will defeat its own ends if it blurs distinctions between methods appropriate for various kinds of learning. Guided drills with attention to form of response will hasten the mastery of skills. Facts will be mastered most thoroughly by attentive association with a multitude of facts already known. Problem solving will be fostered by systematic organization of facts as they are acquired and by arousing curiosity to a high pitch (Tuttle, 1963, p. 294).

Tuttle stated very clearly that some individuals' view of a wholesome philosophy is misapplied in teaching and learning in education.

The format used to develop Modules in this curriculum is as follows:

   I.  Title and number of course

   II.  Title and number of module

   III.  Purpose of module

    IV. Prerequisites

    V. Entry behaviors

    VI. Objectives of module

    VII. Learning activities (including content)

    VIII. Teaching strategies

    IX. Evaluation (including formative and summative)

This format is used throughout the development of courses with some flexibility within the categories. For example, in the first module in the first course in the nursing major, the entry behaviors may be assessed in a different manner than in subsequent modules. Throughout the materials, emphasis is placed on learning and learner rather than on teaching and teacher. Module I is presented in detail as an example.

This module is designed to help students achieve the first objective in the first course in the nursing major. The objectives were written to demonstrate the interrelationship among the cognitive, affective, and psychomotor domains of learning. Also, this is basic knowledge and the beginning of skill learning in perceptual accuracy, in communication skills, in participant and nonparticipant observations, in one-to-one and one-to-group interactions, and in deductive and inductive thinking.

The module objectives are organized under the three knowledge domains. In the cognitive domain, objective 1 is at the level of knowledge, objective 2 is at the level of comprehension, and objectives 3, 4, and 5 are at the level of analysis. In the affective domain, objective 1 is at the level of valuing, and objective 2 is at the high level of characterization of a value. In the psychomotor domain, objectives 1 and 2 indicate ability in two specific skills.

From these behavioral objectives, suggested learning activities are planned for students to practice the behaviors identified in the objectives. When students have had sufficient time to learn the behaviors and have experienced formative evaluation, their achievement of the objectives is determined by summative evaluation.

## NURSING 301   INTRODUCTION TO NURSING

*Module I*

**Title:**   General Systems Framework, A Theory of Goal Attainment, and Observation and Measurement Skills.

**Purpose:**   To introduce students to the conceptual framework that serves as a basis for studying nursing; to help students relate the concepts to growth and development through the life cycle; to introduce students to a systematic way of thinking about their world; and to use a nursing theory of goal attainment.

**Entry Behaviors:**   Junior standing and

1. Complete written examination on selected basic concepts from biophysical sciences, behavioral sciences, and the humanities.

2. Evaluation of students' knowledge of concepts of human interactions and skills in speaking, listening, and writing.

3. Evaluation of verbal and nonverbal behavior in one-to-one and one-to-group interactions.

**Objectives for the Module:**

*Cognitive:*

1. Describe the basic concepts of the framework and a nursing theory of goal attainment.

2. Give examples of basic concepts in situations involving a child, an adolescent, a young adult, and an older adult.

3. Distinguish between facts and inferences in formulating an operational definition of perception, communication, and decision making.

4. Recognize underlying assumptions of the conceptual framework.

5. Recognize human beings and their functional state of health with a focus on a theory of goal attainment.

6. Diagram the interrelationship of the concepts in the conceptual framework and the nursing theory of goal attainment.

*Affective:*

1. Differentiate between inductive and deductive reasoning in developing substantive knowledge of the concepts.

2. Propose a plan for interacting with individuals in a residence for older persons.

*Psychomotor:*

1. Demonstrate skill in verifying perceptual accuracy in role-playing situations in the laboratory.

2. Demonstrate skill in verbal and nonverbal communications, one-to-one and one-to-group in a laboratory situation.

**Content for the Module:**

*Concepts:*

1. Conceptual framework and a theory of goal attainment.

2. Focus of the framework is human–environment interactions.

3. Goal of the system is a functional state of health.

4. Basic concepts of perception, self, body image, growth and development, time, and space in the personal systems.

5. Basic concepts of the interpersonal systems are communication, transaction, interaction, role, and stress.

6. Basic concepts of the social systems are organization, control, status, authority, power, and decision making.

*Skills:*

1. Observation skills as a participant and as a nonparticipant.

2. Communication skills, verbal and nonverbal, and listening and writing.

3. Interview skills using a structured guide.

4. Perceptual skills.

5. Decision-making skills.

*Values:*

1. Rights of human beings.

2. Right to privacy and personal space.

3. Right to participate in events that influence personal growth, development, and performance.

4. Scientific thinking.

**Learning Activities:**

1. Reads about conceptual frameworks and group discussion about their purposes and their basic concepts.

2. Uses a process for developing a concept within this module.

3. Practices observing, recording, and analyzing human behavior related to health across age and socioeconomic groups.

4. Observes and records 15 minutes of a young adult's in-

teraction in a group. Observes and records 15 minutes of an older adult's interaction in a group. Discusses recorded observations with teacher to identify differences between facts and inferences and the value of using an interview guide for systematic collection of information about individuals in different age groups.

5. Uses observation data to differentiate inductive thinking from deductive thinking.

6. Each student begins to develop a concept of perception:

   a. Reviews at least five studies or references in nursing and five references in related fields.

   b. Identifies at least three characteristics of perception and writes a working definition of perception.

   c. Identifies at least two approaches for systematic assessment of an individual's perception of a situation.

   d. Selects two age groups and assesses an individual in each age group; records information and discusses findings with teacher by comparing similarities and differences in perceptions.

   e. Discusses student perceptions, similarities, and differences in recording perceptions of two persons; role plays a situation to verify accuracy of perception of another person.

7. An experience is planned for each student to practice participant and nonparticipant observations in a residence for older individuals.

8. Each experience provides an opportunity for students to practice communications and increase skill in communicating purposefully with individuals to gather relevant information about their health status and health practices.

9. For one week, record the important decisions you made about your life and your health. Discuss with teacher.

10. Note any events in a one-week period in which you thought the rights of human beings were being violated, or the right to privacy ignored, or the right to participate in decisions about individual health accepted or ignored.

11. Discuss the use of a theory of goal attainment in nursing.

**Teaching Strategies:**

1. Mini-lectures to introduce students to new information and to share teacher's concepts related to the theory.

2. Discussion of concepts to help students develop their knowledge.

3. Role playing various communication, interview, and interaction situations using video tapes of behaviors.

4. Demonstrate the participant and nonparticipant observation techniques.

5. Provide structure for direct observations and methods of analyzing data collected.

6. Individual and group conferences between teacher and students.

**Evaluation:**

*Formative:*

1. Conferences with each student and with total group to provide feedback and offer guidance where indicated.

2. Student-initiated conferences for feedback and guidance.

3. First draft of concept paper reviewed by teacher.

4. Analysis of videotape of students' communication, interview, and observations to determine strengths and areas where practice is needed.

*Summative:*

1. Completion of a paper that demonstrates a process for developing concepts of perception, communication, and decision making. Criteria are:

    a. Clarity and consistent format used.

    b. Conciseness.

    c. Identification of at least three characteristics for each concept.

    d. Evidence of analysis of literature.

    e. Minimum of five references in nursing and related fields.

2. Meets all criteria outlined in performance of skills:

    a. Observation data presents reliable information from which inferences can be made and inductive thinking demonstrated.

    b. Perceptions are accurate in at least two different situations recorded.

    c. Skill in verbal communication in at least two situations with two different age groups.

    d. Demonstration of listening skills in at least two situations.

3. A natural situation is presented on videotape that exemplifies the three dynamic, interacting systems of the conceptual framework. Each student must identify at least five basic elements in the situation that influence

health in a positive way. Also, identify at least five behaviors in the situation that may be harmful to health.

The second module introduces students to a concept of
health as the goal for nursing and approaches for systematic
observations and measurements of health status of individuals
and community. This module includes a continuation of skill
learning relative to data collection, facts and inferences, observations, communications, and interactions.

## NURSING 301   INTRODUCTION TO NURSING

### *Module II*

Title:   Health as the Goal for Nursing

Purpose:   To assist students develop a concept of health, skill in
health assessment of individuals, skill in assessment of community health, health-care agencies, values related to health of
human beings, and ethical and legal dimensions and goal attainment.

Prerequisites:   Junior standing and Module I of Nursing 301

Entry Behaviors:

Mastery of Module I of Nursing 301.

Alternate test for summative evaluation for Module I.

Also, submit a one-page paper describing concepts of person, communication, and interactions.

At the beginning of this module, students should be able to:

Cognitive: Relate knowledge from basic and behavioral
sciences and humanities to human–environment interactions.

Affective: Identify three beliefs about health of individuals and community.

Psychomotor: Demonstrate ability to observe and measure individual's perceptions of their health.

**Objectives:** At the completion of this module, students should be able to:

*Cognitive:*

1. Make inferences about human transactions with environment.

2. Apply ethical principles in concrete situations.

3. Identify a minimum of five variables that influence human interactions between individuals and in families relative to a functional state of health.

4. Use a systematic tool to record client's history and health assessment of an adolescent, a young adult, and an older adult.

5. Determine dependency rating in performance of activities of daily living.

6. Identify the characteristics of health.

7. Define health.

8. List a minimum of five laws that govern health in the community, state, and nation.

9. List a minimum of five health indicators.

10. Relate the theory of goal attainment to health as the goal for nursing.

*Affective:*

1. Accept responsibility for personal health practices.

2. Volunteer for community health projects.

3. Recognize that the meaning of health differs from person to person and from society to society.

4. Recognize the importance of accurate perceptions of nurse/client.

*Psychomotor:*

1. Demonstrate skill in gathering information about individuals, groups, and communities.

2. Perform a systematic health assessment of a child and an adult.

3. Demonstrate skill in interviewing and measuring health states of individuals.

4. Verify accuracy of client/nurse perceptions about health status.

**Content of the Module:**

*Concepts:*

Concept of health of individuals, groups, and community.

Concepts of growth and development, role, and stress.

Concepts of time and space.

*Skills:*

1. Assessment which includes observations and measurements of vital signs, history, and health assessment, and measures dependence of individuals.

2. Interview skills.

3. Communication skills.

4. Perceptual accuracy skills.

5. Nursing diagnosis.

*Values:*

1. Right to privacy and to personal space.

2. Right to participate in decisions that affect health.

3. Right to health care with concomitant responsibility to perform health practices.

4  ANA Code for Nurses.

5. ANA Standards of Nursing Care.

6. State laws governing health in the community, state, and nation.

**Learning Activities:**

1. Using assessment guides, observe and record behavior of different ages, sexes, social classes, and social institutions and validate observations.

2. Using a reliable instrument, determine the dependency rating of individuals relative to performance of activities of daily living.

3. Using a systematic form, assess at least one community health agency.

4. Interview individuals of each age group and record their perceptions of their health status. Compare this with your assessment of their health status. Verify accuracy of perceptions of self and those interviewed. Perform a health assessment of an adult.

5. Assess learning needs of individuals to help them maintain their health or prevent illness.

6. Analyze two case studies from real nursing situations related to client rights and the Code for Nurses.

7. Identify at least five laws that govern health in your community, state, and nation.

8. Practice communication skills in the laboratory. Observe and record verbal and nonverbal interactions in a variety of situations and learn the technique of process recording.

9. Practice skills essential for accurate measures of vital signs and physical parameters of individuals.

10. Assess personal health practices and compare differences between own perceptions of health and persons interviewed relative to their health status.

11. Using an assessment tool, gather information about one group of individuals relative to their perceptions of their health status.

12. Observe at least two nurse/client situations, record interactions, and analyze interactions for transactions (King, 1981, pp. 150–151). Determine differences in nurse/client perceptions.

13. Develop a concept of health and submit it for evaluation of knowledge.

14. Develop a concept of growth and development and submit for evaluation of knowledge.

15. Develop a concept of role and stress and submit for evaluation of knowledge.

16. Develop a concept of time and space and submit for evaluation of knowledge.

17. Analyze and discuss the ANA Code for Nurses.

18. Discuss ANA Standards of Nursing Practice.

**Evaluation:**

*Formative:*

1. Teacher and student discuss the consistency between stated ideas about health and health practices and people's behavior related to health practices.

2. Personal perception of health and a concept of health is shared among students and with teacher in large group conferences.

3. First drafts of concept papers are reviewed by teacher and returned to students for guidance and for completion of papers.

4. Direct observation of students conducting assessment and practicing skills in the learning laboratory.

*Summative:*

1. A paper that demonstrates a concept of health.

2. A paper that demonstrates concepts of growth, development, role, stress, time, and space.

3. A paper that demonstrates an objective assessment of one health-care agency in the community.

4. A scrapbook containing current newspaper articles, magazine articles (lay and professional), and health professional studies related to health, law, ethics, and nursing.

5. Performance examination in real nursing situations demonstrating achievement of basic skills such as interviewing, systematic assessment of individuals, communication, and interactions.

6. Given a situation, identify elements that influence decisions related to legal and ethical dimensions of health care.

The objectives to be achieved by students at the completion of Module II are organized sequentially to extend learning achieved in previous experiences. This module provides opportunities for students to increase their assessment skills in the natural environment of a community with relatively healthy individuals. Knowledge of normal ranges in measurements is essential information before students are introduced to more complex types of measurements that show interferences in normal physiology and normal behavior patterns of growth and development.

Modules I and II provide learning experiences for students to grasp the basic knowledge and skills essential for learning to become a professional nurse. Modules I and II have been developed in detail to demonstrate one approach for designing specific modules within specific courses based on a conceptual framework for nursing. These modules are not perfect but are examples of an approach to building comprehensive and complete modules where all elements are interrelated.

The modules demonstrate one approach for developing content in a conceptually-based curriculum as opposed to content that repeats knowledge students should bring from previous courses in other disciplines. When students have developed concepts identified in a curriculum they have gained substantive knowledge, which is what concepts represent. In addition, the process used to develop concepts results in skills in critical analysis and thinking due to practicing inductive and deductive reasoning.

The format used to develop a module assists in completing the first course in the nursing major. The examples of objectives presented in this chapter follow the traditional way of using the taxonomies of educational objectives by Bloom et al. and Krathwohl et al. (1956, 1964). When a faculty group decides to build a compentency-based curriculum, behaviorally stated performance objectives are written. A brief review of this type of objective writing is given for the readers who are moving in this direction.


### Performance Objectives

The characteristics of behavioral objectives have been identified by Mager (1962). He does not seem to agree with Tyler's

(1949) idea that objectives should include behavior and content. Mager suggested that one characteristic of an instructional objective is that it describes behavioral outcome rather than aspects of content.

According to Mager, an objective should be stated in performance terms so that a description of what the learner will be able to do is clear in evaluating the achievement of the objective. A third aspect to this type of objective writing is to describe the conditions under which the behaviors are expected to occur. A fourth dimension is to specify the criteria for judging acceptable performance.

To describe the behavior expected of the learner at the completion of structured experiences, teachers must identify the expected behavioral outcome in the learner related to specific competency criteria, the situation in which the behavior will occur, and the accuracy of the performance. This means that to have a performance objective that is measurable, it must contain the who, which is the noun, and the what, which is the action verb or expected outcome, the how and where, which are the conditions, and the degree of accuracy expected. An example of this may be:

*Objective 1:* Given a list of health indicators, the student identifies at least five that are directly observed or measured in any community 100 percent of the time. This objective contains the who, the student; the what, health indicators; the how, observation or measures; the where, the community; and accuracy, which is 100 percent of the time.

*Objective 2:* Given three individuals to record vital signs of temperature, pulse, respiration, and blood pressure, the student will use appropriate measures and record these signs with 100 percent accuracy.

The objectives above are stated in performance behaviors. The conditions are clearly noted and provide specific criteria for selecting appropriate ways to evaluate student performance.

### Teaching for Specific Learning

If faculty members agree that learning is a change in behavior and behavior is defined as changes in knowledge, changes in skills and changes in values and all of these kinds of learning influence habit formation and attitudes, then curriculum development is influenced by what the faculty members define as essential to learn to become a professional nurse. The structure for the curriculum is a conceptual framework which proposes the organizing elements and guides decision making throughout the process of curriculum development.

A consciously planned approach to teaching will usually bring about effective learning. Deliberative teaching and effective learning are facilitated when a teacher understands at least two kinds of learning. The most dominant kind of behavior in human beings is based on knowledge, which is called conceptual learning or cognition. Conceptual learning is demonstrated when individuals perceive things, have some understanding of their perceptions, view alternatives from which choices can be made about these perceptions, and are able to articulate these ideas. A second kind of learning exhibited in one's behavior is the performance of skills or psychomotor activities. A third kind of learning is values. Learning concepts, which are substantive knowledge, and acquiring of performance abilities, which are psychomotor skills, are two important types of learning essential to become a professional nurse. Entrance into a profession requires learning about the values of that profession and their relationship to an individual's personal values and feelings.

Given knowledge about how individuals learn skills, develop concepts, and acquire values, teachers are in a position to write objectives for modules in courses in a curriculum that are specific, criterion based, and measurable. Accepting the role and functions of a faculty member in higher education requires that nurses seek additional basic preparation in the functional area of teaching.

Research in designing, implementing, and evaluating associate degree programs in community colleges in the 1950's

(Montag, 1951 and 1959) demonstrated the need for faculty preparation beyond the nursing major. A curriculum for an associate degree nursing program is developed in the next chapter.

# A Curriculum
# Leading
# to an
# Associate Degree

The overall aim of an associate degree nursing program is guidance of individuals through planned learning activities to achieve knowledge, skills, values, and attitudes characteristic of a "registered nurse." Upon completion of the program, graduates are able to practice nursing under supervision in selected health-care settings after passing a state licensing examination. A few selected events in the historical development of associate degree nursing programs are highlighted to show some change from the original purpose.

## HISTORICAL DEVELOPMENT OF ASSOCIATE DEGREE PROGRAMS

Programs of study within community colleges have served a variety of functions over the years, such as terminal technical and semi-professional education for occupations, adult education, general education, and community service programs. An initial idea presented a plan for an educational program to prepare nurses to perform technical functions (Montag, 1951). From this initial study followed a five-year curriculum study, experimentation, and evaluation in community college education for nursing, resulting in the development of the associate degree in nursing programs (Montag, 1959). The study demonstrated that individuals could be educated in the two-year program to practice bedside nursing in hospitals. Graduates of the experimental programs performed the functions for which they were prepared, those of direct patient care. Characteristics of associate degree education were published as guiding principles in developing programs (NLNE, 1960). A quotation from this early document indicated that

> graduates of this program are prepared to give patient-centered nursing care in beginning general duty nurse positions. They are prepared to draw upon a background of scientific and humanistic understanding in administering nursing care to patients. They relate well with people and are self directive in learning from experience as practicing nurses. They are prepared to cooperate and share re-

sponsibility for the patients' welfare with other general duty nurses, with head nurses, with supervisors, with attending physicians, and with other personnel. As all other beignning practitioners, these graduates need to be oriented to new work situations and given time and opportunity to become increasingly effective in the practice of nursing (NLNE, 1960, p. 2).

An assumption was made that graduates were not prepared to assume a leadership role at the time of graduation.

After twenty-five years of educating nurses for the technical functions of registered nurses, another set of characteristics was published (NLNE, 1978). The 1960 and 1978 characteristics were similar and no substantive changes in the functions of technical nurses had been made. However, in reviewing some curricula in associate degree nursing programs and the employment requirements in hospitals, changes in nursing care have taken place. For example, critical care units have been established over the years. The nursing care of patients requires advanced knowledge and skills of a highly technical nature. The hospital system for which associate degree graduates were prepared in the past has become so complex in the technology nurses must understand that a beginning staff nurse in hospitals today needs a different kind of preparation than twenty-five years ago. This complex care can only be given and managed by a clinical specialist. The need for nurses prepared for the technical functions related to activities of daily living is still prevalent and has not changed fundamentally from the past.

Quotations from the initial sources for planning associate degree programs are noted here.

The functions of the nurse whose preparation is predominantly technical are: 1) to assist in planning of nursing care for patients, 2) to give general nursing care with supervision, and 3) to assist in evaluation of nursing care given.

In contrast . . . the nurse with professional preparation has responsibilities which are broad in scope. She is responsible for identification and interpretation of nursing problems which are both long term and community wide (Montag, 1951, p. 70).

> The nurse with professional preparation would be able to do all that the nurse with technical preparation does. In addition, she should be able to do those complex activities which are beyond the scope of others concerned with nursing care (Montag, 1951, p. 71).

If this last statement is accepted at face value, there must be some common knowledge and skills required of both the technical and professional nurse. One approach to identify commonalities is to examine the statements of philosophy for the educational programs.

A national survey of philosophies of nursing education has identified some similarities and differences in use of terms (King, 1984). The language used in these statements tells about the beliefs of faculty. Similarities in use of the terms nursing, interpersonal relations, and human beings were found. Differences were in use of terms such as role, perception, social systems, and health. Analysis of the nursing literature implies that there are commonalities in the associate degree and baccalaureate degree programs and the differences are in "breadth" and "depth."

A series of workshops were conducted under the auspices of the NLN to discuss factors that influenced curriculum designs in associate degree programs (DeChow, 1978). In a discussion of associate degree programs, DeChow referred to a curriculum project conducted in the southern region that defined nursing care as primary, secondary, and tertiary. She noted that students in associate degree nursing programs would be taught to function in secondary care settings.

## CHARACTERISTICS OF GRADUATES OF ADN PROGRAMS

The following characteristics were identified by Waters (1978) and published by the NLNE:

1.  "The associate degree graduate defines the client as an individual." The focus is on what the nurse must know to "take care of an individual client, or a group of clients being taken care of as individuals. . . . Generally

speaking, nursing competence of the associate degree graduate is confined to clients who are part of or at home in the dominant culture of the nurse and the health care delivery system" (pp. 6–7).

2. Problems addressed by associate degree graduates are the common and recurring problems of people who seek health care. The problems are "more often physiological than psychological . . ." (p. 7).

3. Intervention in associate degree programs are those "commonly carried out by registered nurses who work with patients who have been diagnosed and are under care in the system." Emphasis is on "responses to problems which are physiological in nature."

4. The context of associate degree nursing practice is in settings in which "nursing services are established and structured. . . . The work setting itself controls the nurses' practice" (p. 8).

5. The "work-world relationships of the associate degree graduate can be characterized as being in a well-defined relationship to the hospital hierarchy, or the hierarchy of the organization in which their work occurs. In addition, associate degree registered nurses are responsible for monitoring and directing the work of others with lesser preparation" (p. 8).

6. "Associate degree graduates' competence in nursing care goals is consistent with knowledge, skills, and attitudes required to care for clients as individuals who have illness problems and the nursing interventions are described, often used, and services are structured and well organized" (p. 8).

These reported characteristics may serve as guidelines for faculty members who are responsible for developing or revising curricula in associate degree nursing programs.

Ideas presented in this book offer one person's point of view on one approach to demonstrate the similarities and differences in associate degree and baccalaureate degree programs in nursing. This approach uses the same conceptual framework for the associate degree nursing program that was used for the baccalaureate program in the previous chapter.

## A HYPOTHETICAL ASSOCIATE DEGREE PROGRAM

The overall purpose of this hypothetical program is the education of individuals to function upon graduation in the role of registered nurses. That role and accompanying functions now and in the future require basic knowledge and skills to provide nursing care in secondary and tertiary care systems of a highly skilled technical nature. These functions are reflected in the society to be served, and this society is demanding highly skilled technical experts in hospitals.

A hypothetical curriculum for an associate degree program in nursing is presented in this chapter. The same elements for developing a curriculum in the last chapter are repeated here and shown in Figure 6.1 to facilitate following the ideas in this chapter.

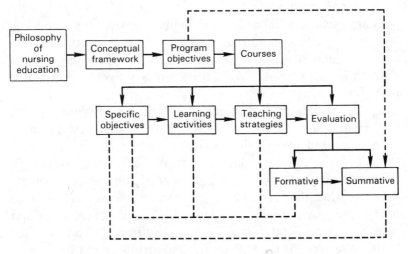

**Figure 6.1**
Curriculum and Instruction Process

The first element states a philosophy of nursing education from which the second element, a conceptual framework, is identified. Subsequent to identification of these elements, objectives are formulated. When agreement of the faculty has been reached about these three elements, courses can be identified. Faculty in associate degree programs in nursing select general education courses that are taken as prerequisites or taken concurrently with nursing courses.

A hypothetical curriculum is proposed to demonstrate the use of ideas in previous chapters. Any resemblance to current programs is purely coincidental.

## Philosophy of Nursing Education

The statement of philosophy for a curriculum in a hypothetical associate degree nursing program is in keeping with the purpose of the community college, democratic society, and the aims of technical nursing. The philosophy is based on assumptions about human beings, society, health, health-care systems, learning, teaching, nursing, and technical nursing education.

Human beings are unique individuals of intrinsic worth who are capable of relating, communicating, thinking, choosing, and making decisions on the basis of their perceptions, background experiences, interests, and goals. Human beings have a right to health care and also a responsibility to engage in health practices.

U.S. society offers citizens the right to freedom, justice, and protection under the Constitution. Social systems have been organized to help individuals achieve goals. Examples of these systems are the family, educational systems, work systems, recreational systems, religious and community organizations, and health-care systems. The social systems are conceived to be the environments within which individuals grow and develop. Local, state, and federal governments provide for health-care systems through public and private sources.

Health care delivery systems have been categorized into primary, secondary, and tertiary care. Ethical and legal issues have been identified that relate to health care of individuals and groups and to the high technology used for treatment and therapy. Secondary care systems, such as hospitals, require highly skilled technical persons in various health occupations. Technical nurses function within these systems under the supervision of a professional nurse or a physician.

Health is defined as the dynamic life experiences of a human being, which implies continuous adjustment to stressors in the internal and external environments through optimum use of one's resources to achieve maximum potential for daily living (King, 1981, p. 5). Initially, health practices are learned within the family.

The primary goal for technical nursing is care of those individuals who are ill and usually hospitalized and care for the dying. Nursing is a human process of interaction between nurse and client within a structured nursing situation. Technical nurses implement the goals identified by the professional nurses and participate in evaluation of goal attainment. Technical nurses function as essential and valued members of the nursing and health team.

Learning is self-activity and requires involvement of individuals in the process. Learning is characterized by thinking and decision making. Learning is an individual experience as each person grows and develops. Each individual has a personal learning style, individual goals, and learns at a different rate of speed. Feedback and reinforcement facilitate learning.

Teaching is a complex process characterized by planning, selecting, assessing, organizing, sequencing, facilitating, guiding, implementing, and evaluating individual learners and programs to achieve goals. A climate is provided for teachers to have the freedom to teach and students to have the freedom to learn. Teaching is goal directed and based on a learner's needs, interests, goals, and program objectives.

Education for technical nursing aims to prepare individuals who are active participants in planned learning activities in a formal education system. Through these activities, individuals learn a systematic way of thinking about nursing and about health care. They gain specific knowledge, skills, and values essential to practice as a technical nurse. In addition, individuals make decisions and act consistently and reasonably as nurses within the occupation of nursing in a democratic society.

The philosophical assumptions serve to guide a faculty group to formulate a framework for the curriculum. The conceptual framework for this associate degree program in nursing follows the theme in this book which is to use a systems approach to curriculum and instruction.

## CONCEPTUAL FRAMEWORK
## FOR THE CURRICULUM

The concepts in the general systems framework used for the baccalaureate program in the previous chapter are used to provide structure for the associate degree curriculum. The concepts in the personal, interpersonal, and social systems are reiterated here for continuity in developing the curriculum.

Personal systems in the diagram relate to each individual. Interpersonal systems are described as dyads, or small and large groups (see p. 117). Social systems are described as those groups that form to achieve specific purposes within a society, such as family, school, business and industry, churches, hospitals, and other health-care organizations. Social systems are the environments within which individuals and groups develop, grow, learn, and perform their functions in life.

Every system has goals. The goal for nursing is health (King, 1971, 1981). However, in the associate degree program, emphasis is placed on care of individuals who are ill, injured and disabled, and care of those who are dying. The aim is to help individuals regain health and if this is not possible, to help them die with dignity. The focus is on helping individuals and providing care for groups of individuals (Waters, 1978, p. 6).

Major concepts are selected within each of the three dynamic interacting systems. A major concept that gives us knowledge about self, about others, and about environment is perception. Concepts related to perception are self, body image, learning, growth, development, time, and space.

A major concept that gives us knowledge about interpersonal systems is human interactions. Concepts related to interaction are communication, transaction, role, and stress. A major concept that gives us knowledge about social systems is organization. Concepts related to organizations are power, control, authority, status, role, and decision making.

An assumption is made that a conceptually designed curriculum assists students gain knowledge and skills for both technical and professional nursing. This assumption is based on Bruner's (1960) concept of a spiral curriculum. Simply explained, a spiral curriculum indicates that common knowledge and skills are required for living in this society. These concepts and skills can be learned at the elementary, secondary, and post-high school level of education. One merely continues to extend knowledge of familiar concepts and to add new knowledge at each level of education. Using the same conceptual framework provides a means for identifying common knowledge and skills in the occupation of nursing. In addition, use of the same conceptual framework provides for articulation from one program to another for those individuals who wish to continue their education.

This framework and the identified concepts provide the structure for the curriculum proposed for educating individuals for technical nursing. From a stated philosophy and conceptual framework, program objectives are formulated.

### Program Objectives

Individuals who select a program of study in a community college should know the outcomes expected of them at the completion of the program. Several factors determine the type of objectives to be achieved to become a technical nurse. Educational standards for entrance into the occupation of nursing are influenced by standards of practice for professional nursing. The following objectives are suggested for a curriculum to prepare technical nurses.

1. Implement nursing care for individuals and groups who are under the supervision of a professional nurse.

2. Use nursing actions to help individuals who are ill return to a functional state of health.

3. Appraise effectiveness of technical aspects of care.

4. Perform functions within secondary health care systems with guidance of a professional nurse.

5. Support the ethical values of professional nursing.

6. Participate as a member of the nursing team to deliver care for individuals and groups.

7. Participate in continuing education to add to knowledge and to increase skills.

8. Perform observations, measurements, and techniques of nursing with accuracy.

A review of the above objectives shows that objective 8 relates to technical skills in nursing and represents the psychomotor domain of knowledge. Knowledge is essential in the practice of technical nursing and objectives 1, 2, 3, and 5 in the cognitive domain are suggested. Objectives 4, 6, and 7 in the affective domain are presented. The importance of the interrelationships between the cognitive and affective domains of knowledge is reflected in the objectives and shows balance. Objectives of this type provide the road map for faculty groups to design a program of study.

From the overall program objectives, which are more general in nature than course objectives, courses are planned by faculty. The program objectives guide faculty both in the selection of courses that provide knowledge from basic and behavioral sciences essential for nursing and in the organization of the nursing courses.

**Prerequisite or Concurrent Courses.** When decisions have been made about the philosophy, conceptual framework, and program objectives, faculty members determine the courses for the program. Courses in areas such as English, sociology, psychology, anatomy, and physiology may be selected to provide students with knowledge from other areas of study. In the community college system courses that cut across disciplines designed for technical programs may be suggested. Examples of such courses are integrated sciences, which include anatomy, physiology, and microbiology; behavioral sciences, which include sociology, psychology, anthropology, political science, economics, and communications.

**Courses in Nursing.** The nursing courses build on knowledge from previous educational experiences. Courses and credit hours for the nursing components of the program are:

| TITLES | CREDIT HOURS |
|---|---|
| Introduction to Nursing | 3 |
| Practicum in Introduction to Nursing | 3 |
| Nursing Skills Laboratory | 2 |
| Nursing of Individuals | 6 |
| Practicum in Nursing of Individuals | 6 |
| Nursing of Individuals in Groups | 6 |
| Practicum in Nursing of Individuals in Groups | 6 |
| Role and Functions in Technical Nursing | 2 |
| Practicum in Performing Functions in Role of Technical Nurse | 4 |
| Issues and Trends in Nursing | 3 |

Forty-one credit hours are suggested for meeting the requirements for nursing in this associate degree program.

Attention is given to sequence when faculty groups select courses and plan for instruction. Sequence means that teachers believe that prior knowledge and skills are essential before learners can move on to new activities. Piaget's studies of the intellectual development of children, Bruner's ideas about the structure of subject matter in a curriculum, and Bloom and colleagues' studies and publications support the idea of sequence as a major component in organizing a curriculum to facilitate student learning.

## Placement of Courses in the Curriculum

| FIRST YEAR | CREDIT HOURS |
|---|---|
| *First Semester* | |
| Introduction to Human Anatomy and Physiology | 4 |
| History | 3 |
| Developmental Psychology | 2 |
| Nursing Skills Laboratory | 2 |
| Introduction to Nursing | 2 |
| Practicum in Introduction to Nursing | 3 |
| *Second Semester* | |
| Literature | 3 |
| Human Communications | 2 |
| Developmental Psychology | 2 |
| Introduction to Microbiology | 3 |
| Nursing of Individuals | 2 |
| Practicum in Nursing Care of Individuals | 3 |
| Skills in Nursing of Individuals | 2 |

| SECOND YEAR | CREDIT HOURS |
|---|---|
| *First Semester* | |
| Art Appreciation | 2 |
| Music Appreciation | 2 |
| Nursing Care of Individuals in Groups | 4 |
| Practicum in Care of Groups | 6 |
| Skills in Nursing Care of Groups | 2 |
| *Second Semester* | |
| Ethical and Legal Perspectives in Technical Nursing | 3 |
| Role and Functions in Technical Nursing | 4 |
| Practicum in Functioning in Role of Technical Nurse | 6 |
| Issues and Trends in Nursing | 3 |

None of the above courses are developed in detail in this book; however, examples are given to demonstrate the use of a conceptual approach to curriculum and instruction. When faculty members have made decisions about the nursing courses to be taught and the sequence in which learners will enroll in the courses, a format for instructional planning, shown in Figure 6.2, is repeated to maintain a flow of ideas.

The process begins first with formulation of objectives for each course in terms of behavior outcomes in the cognitive, affective, and psychomotor domains. Second, selections of learning activities are made so students can practice the behaviors they are expected to achieve. Third, teaching strategies are selected that will provide guidance, feedback, and reinforcement for learners. Fourth, learning materials related to objectives are prepared. Fifth, formative evaluation is a process of feedback for corrective action by learners, if necessary. This process is an ongoing teacher function during the learning process to facilitate learning. Summative evaluation is planned and time established for the teacher to evaluate the learner's achievement of the objective. This evaluation is used for grading in a system that requires a grade at the completion of a module or course.

For purposes of illustration, one course in this hypothetical curriculum will be developed. Two modules in the course will be developed in detail to demonstrate the relation of the instruc-

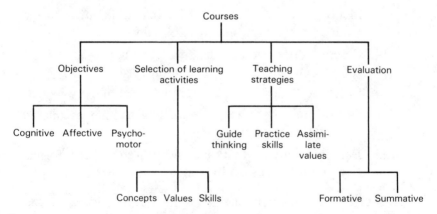

**Figure 6.2**
Instructional Process

tional process outlined in Figure 6.3 to program objectives, conceptual framework and philosophy.

A format is used to show one approach for preparing course materials. The title and number of the course is Nursing 101, Introduction to Nursing. The format begins with a course description.

**Course Description:**   A general systems framework for nursing is emphasized in which concepts of perception, self, body image, communication, interactions, transactions, health, environment, and activities of daily living are developed. Skills in observation, measurement of activities of daily living, and vital signs are acquired. (A note is made here that the second skills course emphasizes communications, interactions, transactions, and perception to correlate with knowledge from courses taken in the college.)

**Course Objectives:**   At the completion of this course, students will be able to:

1. Outline a general systems framework for the curriculum.

2. Distinguish between facts and inferences in gathering data from observations and measurements of client's health status.

3. Identify the dependency of a client from each age group in performing activities of daily living.

4. Describe differences in the perceptions of an adolescent and an older adult about health practices.

5. Demonstrate health practices in activities of daily living.

6. Demonstrate skills in basic nursing techniques related to activities of daily living.

7. Demonstrate use of an objective tool to gather information about client's health status.

The course objectives were planned to introduce students to the framework of the curriculum and its relationship to nursing.

An approach to cross check the way course objectives help learners achieve program objectives is shown in Figure 6.3. The

NURSING 101 COURSE OBJECTIVES

| PROGRAM OBJECTIVES | Nr. 101 INTRODUCTION to NURSING | Nr. 102 PRACTICUM I INTRO. to Nr. |
|---|---|---|
| Implement nursing care for individuals and groups who are under the supervision and care of a professional nurse. | X | |
| Use nursing actions to help individuals who are ill return to a functional state of health. | | X |
| Appraise the effectiveness of technical aspects of care. | X | X |
| Perform functions within secondary health care systems with guidance of a professional nurse. | | X |
| Support the ethical values of professional nursing. | | |
| Participate as a member of the nursing team to deliver effective care for individuals and groups. | | |
| Participate in continuing education to add to knowledge and to increase skills. | | |
| Skill in performing with accuracy observations, measurements, and techniques of nursing. | | X |

**Figure 6.3**

Relationship of Program Objectives to Course
Objectives

course objectives and the module objectives are written to provide specific opportunities in the cognitive, affective, and psychomotor domains of learning. For example, in the course proposed here, objectives 1, 2, and 3 are cognitive; objectives 4 and 5 are affective; and objectives 6 and 7 are psychomotor. The objectives are written to show relationships which facilitate faculty members' choice of learning activities. From course objectives, the objectives for each module are written to help students achieve the course objectives. For the first nursing course in the hypothetical curriculum for an associate degree program, the modules are identified as follows:

Module 1. General systems framework and introduction to observation and measurement skills.

Module 2. Health as a goal.

Module 3. Personal systems are individuals and groups are called interpersonal systems.

Module 4. Basic skills for technical nursing.

Module 5. Concepts of perception, learning, self, and body image.

Module 6. Concepts of human interactions and stress.

Module 7. Social systems as environment.

Module 8. Local and state morbidity and mortality statistics.

The first module introduces students to the course, teachers' expectations of learners, and learners' expectations of teachers. Each module is organized to let the students know the overall course and then to learn concepts, process, and skills in this first course as a basis for requirements in the courses that help them achieve a goal of becoming a highly skilled technical nurse.

The first two modules are developed in detail and the same format is used to develop the remaining modules. The ideas presented in the first two modules are an approach to demonstrate a conceptually-based course in a nursing curriculum in an associate degree program. The difference between this course for this program and the same type of course for the baccalaureate program is the base of knowledge, which is more comprehensive in the baccalaureate curriculum. The process for developing concepts can be found in several sources (King, 1975, 1981). Students are provided with a selected bibliography to help them begin to develop certain concepts. However, teachers provide knowledge about the concepts in the teaching materials rather than students having to develop all of the concepts themselves.

Students in the associate and baccalaureate programs are expected to use the nursing process as defined by Yura and Walsh (1983). In using this process the differences between the two curricula are in the knowledge base and in critical thinking related to gathering facts, making inferences, and identifying goals to be achieved.

Students are introduced to the overall framework of the program in the first module in the first course in nursing. This gives them an overview of the total curriculum and expectations for achievement in the program.

The format used to develop modules in this curriculum is as follows:

    I. Title and number of course

    II. Title and number of module.

    III. Purpose of module

    IV. Prerequisites

    V. Entry behaviors

    VI. Objectives of the module

    VII. Learning activities (including content)

    VIII. Teaching strategies

    IX. Evaluation (including formative and summative)

This format is used throughout the development of courses with some flexibility within the categories. For example, in the first module in the first course in nursing, the entry behaviors may be assessed in a different manner than in subsequent modules. Throughout the materials, emphasis is placed on learning and learner rather than teaching and teacher. Module I is presented in detail as an example.

## NURSING 101   INTRODUCTION TO NURSING

*Module I*

**Title:**   General Systems Framework and Introduction to Observation and Measurement Skills

**Purpose:**   To introduce students to the conceptual framework of the curriculum; to help students relate the concepts of growth and development through the life cycle; to introduce students to a systematic way of gathering objective information about clients.

**Entry Behaviors:**

1. Written examination on selected basic concepts related to health and health practices of all age and sociocultural groups.

2. Evaluation through selected situations of the student's knowledge of human interactions and skills in speaking, writing, and listening.

3. Evaluation of verbal and nonverbal behavior in one-to-one and one-to-group interactions.

**Objectives for the Module:**

*Cognitive:*

1. Demonstrate beginning knowledge of the basic concepts of the framework related to individuals.

2. Explain procedures for gathering facts and making inferences as a basis for planning nursing care of individuals.

3. Relate information gathered to the health or illness of individuals.

*Affective:*

4. Explain differences between growth and development in each age group.

5. Describe the relationship between perception, learning, and body image.

*Psychomotor:*

6. Ability to follow a procedure in observing and recording health practices in an adult and a child.

7. Skill in use of a reliable tool to assess a client's health status.

### Content for the Module:

*Concepts:*

1. A conceptual framework.

2. Goal of technical nursing is to help clients regain health following illness and disability.

3. Basic knowledge of concepts of perception, self, body image, growth and development, and time and space in personal systems.

4. Basic concepts of human–environment interaction and stress.

5. Basic concepts of social systems are organization, control, status, authority, power, and decision making.

*Skills:*

1. Observation skills using a structured guide.

2. Interview skills using a structured guide.

3. Measurement of vital signs of temperature, blood pressure, pulse, and respiration.

4. Basic nursing techniques related to activities of daily living.

*Values:*

1. Rights of human beings.

2. Right to privacy.

3. Right to participate in events that influence personal growth, development, and performance.

### Learning Activities:

1. Selected readings on each of the concepts in this module. Develop in detail a concept of perception, human interactions, growth, and development using a process.

2. Practice observing and recording human interactions in one-to-one and one-to-group activities of all age levels and across socioeconomic groups.

3. Discuss recorded observations with teacher to identify differences between facts and inferences and the value of using structured guides for accuracy and objectivity.

4. Practice measurements of vital signs in laboratory and seek formative evaluation from teacher.

5. For one week, record the important decisions you made about your life and your health. Discuss with teacher decision making and consequences of decisions.

6. Note any events in a one-week period in which you thought the rights of human beings were being violated; the right to privacy ignored; or the right to participate in decisions about individual health accepted or ignored.

**Teaching Strategies:**

1. Lecture and discussion to introduce students to concepts and the process for developing them.

2. Group discussions of all concepts in the framework.

3. Role play various interview and interaction situations.

4. Demonstrate structured interview techniques and structured observations of individuals.

5. Individual and group conferences between teacher and students.

**Evaluation:**

*Formative:*

1. Conferences with each student and with total group to provide feedback and offer guidance when indicated.

2. Student-initiated conferences for feedback and guidance.

3. First draft of concept paper reviewed by teacher.

4. Analyze videotape of students' interview and observation techniques.

*Summative:*

1. Completion of a paper that demonstrates beginning development of three concepts. Criteria are:

   a. Clarity and consistent format.

   b. Conciseness.

   c. Identification of at least three characteristics for each concept developed.

   d. Evidence of reading in nursing and related fields.

2. Meets all criteria outlined in performance of skills:

   a. Performs measures of temperature, blood pressure, pulse, and respiration with 100 percent accuracy in at least three natural situations.

   b. Gathers reliable information about health status from a structured interview in at least two natural situations, one with a child and one with an adult.

   c. Perceptions are accurate in a dyadic interaction with an adolescent and an older adult.

   d. A natural situation is presented on videotape that exemplifies the three dynamic interacting systems of the conceptual framework. Each student must identify at least three elements in the situation that influences health in a positive way. Also, identify at least three elements in the situation that may be harmful to health.

This module is designed to help students achieve the first objective in the first course in nursing. The objectives were written to demonstrate the interrelationship between cognitive, affective, and psychomotor domains of learning. Also, this is basic knowledge and the beginning of skill learning in observations and measurements of health status. Figure 6.4 shows the relationship between the module objectives and the course objectives. This format was borrowed from Tyler (1949, p. 50).

In the cognitive domain, objectives 1, 2, and 3 are at the level of comprehension, application, and synthesis. In the affective domain, objectives 4 and 5 are at the level of valuing. In the psychomotor domain, objectives 5 and 6 indicate ability in two specific skills. From these behavioral objectives, suggested learning activities are planned for students to practice the behaviors identified in the objectives. When students have had sufficient time to learn the behaviors and have experienced formative evaluation, their achievement of the objectives is determined by summative evaluation.

NURSING 101

| Course Objectives | Module Objectives | | | | | | | |
|---|---|---|---|---|---|---|---|---|
| | 1 | 2 | 3 | 4 | 5 | 6 | 7 | 8 |
| Outline a general systems framework for the curriculum | X | X | X | X | X | X | X | X |
| Distinguish between facts and inferences in gathering data from observations and measurements of clients health status. | | | X | X | X | X | | X |
| Identify the dependency of a client from each age group in performing activities of daily living. | | | X | X | X | X | X | X |
| Describe differences in the perceptions of an adolescent and an older adult about health practices. | | X | X | X | X | X | X | |
| Demonstrate health practices in activities of daily living. | | X | X | X | X | | X | X |
| Demonstrate skill in basic nursing techniques related to activities of daily living. | | X | X | X | X | X | X | X |
| Demonstrate use of an objective tool to gather information about clients health status. | | X | X | X | X | X | | |

**Figure 6.4**

Relationship between Course Objectives and Module Objectives

The second module introduces students to a concept of health as a goal for nursing with emphasis on relatively healthy clients as a basis for learning about interferences in health status of individuals. This module includes a continuation of skill learning relative to data collection, facts and inferences, observations and measurements. Emphasis will be given to communications and human interactions.

## NURSING 101 INTRODUCTION TO NURSING

*Module II*

**Title:** Health as a Goal for Nursing

**Purpose:** To assist students develop a concept of health, skill in health assessment of individuals, and values related to health of human beings with initial emphasis on ethical and legal dimensions of health care.

**Prerequisites:** Module I of Nursing 101

**Entry Behaviors:**

Mastery of Module I of Nursing 101.

Alternate test for summative evaluation for Module I.

Also, each student submits a one-page paper describing concepts of person, human interactions, and perception.

At the beginning of this module, students should be able to:

Cognitive: Relate knowledge of self, perception, and body image to healthy individuals; demonstrate beginning skill in observation and selected measures, such as vital signs.

Affective: Identify three factors that may be harmful to health and three factors that promote health.

Psychomotor: Determine accuracy of perceptions between nurse and client in three natural situations.

**Objectives:** At the completion of this module, students should be able to:

*Cognitive:*

1. List at least three laws that govern health in your community and state.

2. Identify two situations in which you think an indi-

vidual's privacy was preserved and two in which privacy was violated.

3. Rate the dependency of an older person and of a child in performance of activities of daily living.

4. Use a structured interview guide to assess the health status of an adolescent and an adult.

5. Define your concept of health.

*Affective:*

1. Accept responsibility for personal health practices.

2. Recognize the differences in individuals' perception of health.

3. Volunteer for at least one community health project.

*Psychomotor:*

1. Demonstrate skill in gathering reliable information about the health status of selected individuals.

2. Demonstrate skill in measuring at least five parameters of health states in individuals.

3. Verify the accuracy of your perceptions with two client's perceptions of health status.

**Content of the Module:**

*Concepts:*

Concept of health of individuals.

Concept of growth and development of individuals.

Concept of role of individuals in society, such as child, adolescent, young adult, and older adult.

Concept of stress related to health status.

Concept of time and space.

*Skills:*

1. Observation of vital signs and measure of dependence of individuals.

2. Purposeful communication skills.

3. Human interactions skills.

*Values:*

1. Right to privacy.

2. Right to health care with concomitant responsibility to perform health practices.

3. ANA Code for Nurses.

4. Nursing diagnosis.

5. Local and state laws governing health.

### Learning Activities

1. Using an interview guide, observe and record health behaviors of a child, an adolescent, and a young adult.

2. Using a reliable scale, determine the dependency rating of three individuals relative to performance of activities of daily living.

3. Assess learning needs of three individuals who need assistance in maintaining their health and managing a chronic disease.

4. Analyze at least two case studies related to application of the Code for Nurses.

5. Practice skills essential for accurate measures of vital signs and physical parameters of individuals' health status.

6. Practice purposeful interactions with a child and an adult.

7. Interview five individuals in the community to determine their knowledge of health practices.

8. Develop your concept of health, growth and development, stress, time and space, and submit for evaluation of your knowledge.

**Evaluation:**

*Formative:*

1. Teacher and student discuss the similarities and differences between stated ideas about health and health practices and individual behavior related to health practices.

2. Personal perception of health and a concept of health is shared among students and with teacher in large group conferences.

3. First drafts of concept papers are reviewed by teacher and returned to student for guidance and for completion of papers.

4. Direct observation of students conducting interviews, assessments of vital signs, and practicing other skills in the laboratory.

*Summative:*

1. Papers that demonstrate personal concept of health, growth and development, stress, and time and space.

2. A paper that summarizes your perceptions of persons interviewed about their health status.

3. A scrapbook containing at least three current newspaper articles, magazine articles (lay and professional), and studies related to health, at least one legal and one ethical dimension of nursing and health care.

4. Performance examination demonstrating achievement of basic skills such as interviewing, interactions, observations, and measurements of individuals relative to their health status.

5. Performance examination demonstrating skill in assessing individual's abilities to perform activities of daily living.

The objectives to be achieved by students at the completion of Module II are organized sequentially to extend learning achieved in previous experiences. This module provides opportunities for students to increase their assessment skills with relatively healthy individuals. Knowledge of normal ranges in measurements is essential information before students are introduced to more complex measures that show interferences in human behavior patterns.

Modules I and II provide learning experiences for students to grasp the basic knowledge and skills essential for learning to become a technical nurse. Modules I and II have been developed in detail to demonstrate one approach for designing specific modules within specific courses based on a conceptual framework for nursing. These modules are neither perfect nor completely developed but are examples of an approach to building comprehensive and complete modules where all elements are interrelated.

The modules demonstrate one approach for developing content in a conceptually based curriculum as opposed to content that repeats knowledge students should bring from previous courses and past experiences. When students have developed concepts or learned the substantive knowledge of a concept from others, they have gained substantive knowledge, which is what concepts represent. In addition, the process used by students to develop substantive knowledge helps them learn how to think logically.

When a faculty group decides to develop a competency-based curriculum, behaviorally stated performance objectives are written. An example of this type of objective was given in the previous chapter and a reference to Mager given for those who want to develop this type of objective. The last chapter also provided sources for learning how to teach for specific kinds of learning, such as concept learning and skill learning.

Attention is called to the fact that the two modules in the first course in nursing in the associate degree and baccalaureate degree programs are similar. The differences are in the knowledge the baccalaureate students bring to the first course from two years of study in basic sciences, behavioral sciences, and the humanities, and in experiences in critical thinking and decision making. In other courses, learning experiences for students in each of the two programs differ in knowledge, skills, and scientific thinking in making transactions through purposeful communications to identify goals and implement the means to achieve those goals for individuals who need nursing care.

The next chapter will discuss one approach for trying to resolve the problems of articulation between associate degree and baccalaureate degree programs.

# chapter 7

# Articulation Between ADN* and BSN** Programs

*ADN—Associate Degree in Nursing.
**BSN—Bachelor of Science in Nursing.

For many years, individuals have identified one or more problems in advancing themselves educationally, especially in seeking admission to colleges and universities. They ask questions such as, "Why don't I receive credit for my previous education?", "Why don't I receive credit for my experience?", "Why didn't the high school counselor give me accurate information about nursing programs?", and "Why can't continuing education programs be given credit toward a bachelor of science degree?"

Many more questions have been asked about the problem of articulation from one educational program to another. The problem of articulation between ADN and BSN programs has been discussed in the nursing literature and at professional meetings for years. Some nurse educators have advocated a ladder concept while others have rejected it. Faculty members in some programs have implemented ideas that have solved individual admission problems. Very little has been written about solving the problem through purposefully designed curricula. This chapter presents one approach, if implemented, to solve the problem. In addition, for those individuals who reject the idea of articulation, ideas are presented and questions raised about this approach to curriculum development.

## OVERVIEW OF THE PROBLEM IN NURSING

In the early part of the twentieth century, junior colleges were established in some parts of the United States to provide the first two years of education for transfer to senior colleges and universities. This single-purpose institution was modified following World War II when an educational movement to establish community colleges in each state was implemented.

Research and development in the early 1950's generated increased knowledge in many fields of study and increased technology in industry and in health-care systems. This increase in technology and knowledge continues to bombard us in all areas of living. This brought forth a need to provide two years of post-secondary education to train persons for highly skilled occupations, to prepare technicians to work in the new jobs that were being created. These changes in society brought about changes in the educational system and influenced nursing education.

Studies and reports in nursing and nursing education since the early part of the twentieth century have recommended changes in the nursing education system. The one change most often suggested was to place education for nursing within the general system of education in the United States (Brown, 1948; ANA, 1965; ANA, 1978). At the time of the community college movement, a nurse completed a doctoral study that recommended education for nurses within community colleges. These programs would prepare individuals for the functions identified at that time as those of the "registered nurse."

A five-year study was conducted from 1952 to 1957 which demonstrated that a two-year curriculum in a community college could prepare individuals to function as registered nurses (Montag, 1959). The results of the study indicated that nursing education can take place in community colleges. Following this research and demonstration project, associate degree programs in nursing increased at a phenomenal rate.

Many articles and studies have been reported in nursing journals and in books about the associate degree nursing curriculum, about the graduates of these programs, and about the problems confronting nursing education's system for the rest of the twentieth century. Similar studies of baccalaureate programs have not been reported. However, a few studies have been conducted within single university programs that demonstrated curriculum revision and changes.

Several problems have been discussed relative to articulation between ADN and BSN programs. For example, faculty members who develop an ADN curriculum make decisions about basic and behavioral science courses essential for the program. If the group decides to select "general education" courses for the requisites for the nursing curriculum rather than specific courses that are considered as "transfer" courses, this may present a problem in using these credits for admission to baccalaureate programs. Another problem is that of preparing individuals in a specific curriculum to become socialized into a role, such as the professional role of a nurse. A philosophical problem cited by some individuals is that the ADN program is not the basis for the BSN program. Montag (1951) noted that professional nurses must be able to do all that the nurse with technical preparation does, and in addition perform complex activities beyond the scope of other nursing personnel (p. 71). Does this assume that there are some commonalities in the two programs?

All of the problems mentioned are real for those individuals involved. However, in light of new information from studies in learning, education, curriculum development, and learner evaluations, the 1980's may be a time when nursing educators could exert leadership in curriculum development in higher education. One approach is the development of curricula that solve the problem of articulation.

## A RATIONALE TO FACILITATE ARTICULATION

One approach for designing curricula for nursing education to facilitate articulation from an associate degree to a baccalaureate degree program is presented. The rationale for this approach is based on three major events in education the past twenty years. These events are: 1) Bruner's concept of a spiral curriculum and the structure of a subject; 2) a concept of mastery learning; and 3) assessment of learners' knowledge and performance through diagnostic, formative, and summative evaluation of learners.

**Spiral Curriculum.** In the late 1950's a variety of curriculum projects were being conducted related to teaching science in elementary and secondary schools in the United States. Through the efforts and support of many individuals and several agencies, a conference of educators, scientists, educational media experts, and those conducting the curriculum projects was held in 1959. The chairman of the planning committee also compiled the results of the deliberations of experts who attended the conference (Bruner, 1960). Several themes were mentioned in this report. One, the structure of a subject, is useful in looking at the problem of articulation.

The fundamental structure of subjects and the role of structure in learning provided insight into curriculum development and instruction. Another theme at the conference was "readiness for learning." One statement that has been frequently quoted—"the foundation of any subject may be taught to anybody at any age in some form" (Bruner, 1960, p. 12)—is helpful in analyzing the fundamental structure of a subject.

A concept of a spiral curriculum was mentioned in the Bruner report of the conference. It was defined as "a curriculum that turns back on itself at each level of education" (Bruner, 1960, p. 13). Bruner noted that a curriculum should be built around the relevant knowledge, skills, and values that are of concern in perpetuating a society. These ideas can be organized in a curriculum to introduce children at an early age to the ideas deemed essential in a society. He proposed that a curriculum should present the basic ideas of a subject repeatedly, building on them until learners have truly learned the subject. This is similar to developing the basic concepts of a discipline. One gains knowledge of the basic and general ideas of a subject, moves to principles and laws, and then to the applicability of this knowledge to new problems in the future.

The problem in curriculum development has been how to restructure subjects and learning materials so students of different backgrounds and abilities can learn. When learners are able to transfer knowledge learned in previous experiences to new and different situations and add to that knowledge, they have some continuity in learning. *Part of the articulation problem is that curricula have not been structured to introduce learners to the basic ideas of the subject.* Knowledge, acquired as facts or bits and pieces of information, is likely to be forgotten if not acquired within some kind of structure. "To learn the structure of a subject is to know how things are related" (Bruner, 1960, p. 7). This idea has some relation to a concept of mastery learning.

**Mastery Learning.**   A concept of mastery learning was discussed in Chapter 1.   The work of Carroll (1963) and Bloom et al. (1971) has demonstrated a more efficient and economical way to conduct an educational system that facilitates learning. Criterion-referenced evaluation rather than norm-referenced evaluation measures an individual learner's achievement of objectives. The focus is on guiding individual learning.

Mastery learning is based on aptitude, which is the amount of time required to master specific learning tasks, on specific learning activities related to objectives, and on instruction related to student learning styles. All students can master learning tasks if they persevere in time spent in learning. The quality of the instruction and provisions for formative evaluation throughout the learning process provides feedback and reinforcement to help students master the tasks (Carroll, 1963).

A key factor in mastery learning is the determination by teachers of the learners' previous knowledge and skills. This requires diagnostic evaluation prior to beginning new learning experiences. If students do not have the prerequisite knowledge or skills, it will be difficult for them to master new learning tasks.

Another factor is the preparation of adequate learning activities specifically related to the objectives. Another element in implementing a concept of mastery learning in a curriculum is the need for formative evaluation throughout the learning process. Summative evaluation provides information as to whether or not students have achieved mastery in a module or a course. Evaluation is an important part of implementing mastery learning.

**Evaluation.** A comprehensive view of formative and summative evaluation of learners was presented by Bloom and colleagues (1971). Evaluation was defined as "the systematic collection of evidence to determine whether, in fact, certain changes are taking place in the learners as well as to determine the amount or degree of changes in individual students" (Bloom et al., 1971, p. 8). Education is a process which purposefully changes learners as they pass through a curriculum in a school system and have received instruction from teachers. Some changes in students can be attributed to maturation in the process of growth and development. Some changes are influenced by a variety of experiences in groups outside the educational system. Also, within the educational system, students are influenced positively or negatively by specific teachers, by interactions among students, teachers, and administrators, by subjects studied, and by a combination of any of these experiences.

Teachers are responsible for decisions about the changes expected in learners. One kind of decision usually made by teachers and shared with students is the establishment of objectives. In some educational situations, teachers and students mutually set goals to be achieved. A prevalent belief exists that teachers are responsible for making explicit the changes expected in students as early as possible in a unit of study, course, or total program.

The structure of the learning process comprises several components. First, objectives to be achieved by learners are stated. This provides direction for the instructional process in terms of outcomes expected in learners at the completion of the program.

Second, diagnostic evaluation of the learners at the beginning of the module or course is done to determine if students have the necessary prerequisites for entering the learning situation. The results provide information in guiding learners through a series of learning activities.

Third, the instructional process, which includes formative evaluation of learners, guides them in acquiring knowledge and skills leading to changes in behavior. Formative evaluation has been defined as an evaluation of student learning during a module or course, and if necessary, changes are made on the basis of current attainment of objectives.

Summative evaluation of learners designates student achievement at the end of a course or module "when no subsequent changes in instruction for that learning will be made" (Bloom et al., 1971, p. 262). Table 7.1 shows the similarities and differences between diagnostic, formative and summative evaluation (Bloom et al., 1971, pp. 91–92).

Three important types of evaluation have been used to assess learners' knowledge and skills. Diagnostic evaluation is conducted prior to entry into a new learning experience or a new educational program. Formative evaluation is conducted during the learning experiences to guide students. Summative evaluation is conducted at the completion of a module, course, or program to determine attainment of objectives.

*Diagnostic evaluation* is used to determine prerequisite knowledge and skills for students to begin a new series of learning experiences in a curriculum. The major purpose of this type of evaluation is to place the student in an appropriate sequence of learning experiences in a curriculum. Those who show they have attained the prerequisites may move on to the next experience. Those who do not exhibit attainment of the objectives may become discouraged and may not be successful in subsequent experiences. For example, in nursing, a student who has not mastered the basic skills required to measure vital signs of patients admitted to hospitals would find it difficult, if not impossible, to complete a health assessment of patients, since the skill of measuring blood pressure, pulse, temperature, and respiration is a part of the assessment.

One of the problems in nursing curricula is that few programs use diagnostic evaluation to determine student achievement of prerequisite learning. This is an area of research in nursing education that is long overdue. The expansion of a concept of diagnostic evaluation in this book is not possible, but references are suggested for readers interested in working on this problem in nursing education.

*Formative evaluation* was initially used in the implementation of a new curriculum to gather evidence and make revisions. Formative evaluation has become useful in guiding students through learning experiences without the anxiety of grading. Teachers are in a position to gather information about student achievement in the process of their learning and attainment of behavior changes. One evaluation approach that may be of assistance for teachers is the use of the CIPP (context, input, process, product) model (Stufflebeam, 1971). The use of this model was demonstrated by Steele (1978) to "systematically evaluate a graduate program in Child Health Nursing leading to a Master of Science degree" (Steele, 1978, p. xi). This model is designed to gather evidence about the construction and imple-

**TABLE 7.1**

Similarities and Differences between Diagnostic,
Formative, and Summative Evaluation

| | TYPE OF EVALUATION | | |
| --- | --- | --- | --- |
| | DIAGNOSTIC | FORMATIVE | SUMMATIVE |
| Function | Placement: Determining the presence or absence of prerequisite skills | Feedback to student and teacher on student progress through a unit | Certification or grading of students at the end of a unit, semester, or course |
| | Determining the student's prior level of mastery | Location of errors in terms of the structure of a unit so that remedial alternative instruction techniques can be prescribed | |
| | Classifying the student according to various characteristics known or thought to be related to alternative modes of instruction | | |
| | Determination of underlying causes of repeated learning difficulties | | |

184

| | | | |
|---|---|---|---|
| Time | For placement at the outset of a unit, semester, or year's work<br><br>During instruction when student evidences repeated inability to profit fully from ordinary instruction | During instruction | At the end of a unit, semester, or year's work |
| Emphasis in evaluation | Cognitive, affective, and psychomotor behaviors<br><br>Physical, psychological, and environmental factors | Cognitive behaviors | Generally cognitive behaviors; depending on subject matter; sometimes psychomotor; occasionally affective behaviors |
| Type of instrumentation | Formative and summative instruments for pretests<br><br>Standardized achievement tests<br><br>Standardized diagnostic tests<br><br>Teacher-made instruments<br><br>Observation and checklists | Specially designed formative instruments | Final or summative examinations |

**TABLE 7.1** *(cont.)*

Similarities and Differences between Diagnostic, Formative, and Summative Evaluation

| | TYPE OF EVALUATION | | |
|---|---|---|---|
| | DIAGNOSTIC | FORMATIVE | SUMMATIVE |
| How objectives of evaluation are sampled | Specific sample of each pre-requisite entry behavior | Specific sample of all re-lated tasks in the hier-archy of the unit | A sample of weighted course objectives |
| | Sample of weighted course objectives | | |
| | Sample of student vari-ables hypothesized or known to be related to a particular type of instruction | | |
| | Sample of physically, emotionally, or environ-mentally related behaviors | | |

| | | | |
|---|---|---|---|
| Item difficulty | Diagnosis of prerequisite skills and abilities: a large number of easy items, 65% difficulty or higher | Cannot be specified beforehand | Average difficulty, ranging from 35% to 70%, with some very easy and some very difficult items |
| Scoring | Norm- and criterion-referenced | Criterion-referenced | Generally norm-referenced but can be criterion-referenced |
| Method of reporting scores | Individual profile by subskills | Individual pattern of pass-fail scores on each task in the hierarchy | Total score or subscores by objectives |

*Source:* B.S. Bloom, J.T. Hastings, and G.F. Madaus, *Handbook on Formative and Summative Evaluation.* New York: McGraw Hill, 1971, p. 91.

mentation of a curriculum, about entry behaviors, and about making changes during implementation of the curriculum or of a course within it to facilitate the teaching–learning process and the attainment of objectives.

*Summative evaluation* is used at the completion of a module or course for assigning a grade. It is directed toward assessment of learner achievement of objectives. The general procedure for constructing test items can be learned in the excellent books written for that purpose (see "References").

The three major elements discussed in this chapter, a concept of a spiral curriculum, a concept of mastery learning, and the three types of evaluation, have been discussed in the curriculum literature for at least the past twenty years. These ideas serve as a rationale for articulation of the associate degree and baccalaureate degree programs in nursing in higher education.

## A SPIRAL CURRICULUM IN NURSING

The structure of the subject called nursing has been defined in several publications (Torres and Yura, 1974; King, 1981; ANA, 1980; Fawcett, 1984). The disciplinary matrix for nursing has been described as open systems of individuals and groups interacting with environments of a physical and social nature. The major concepts of this structure are human beings, health, environment, and nursing. Within these major concepts, examples of subconcepts have been identified and described, such as self, perception, communication, growth, development, performance of activities of daily living, time, personal space, role, and stress. A spiral curriculum indicates that the major concepts and subconcepts are the basis for identifying objectives and related content in developing curricula for nursing at every level of education, from associate degree programs to baccalaureate programs to graduate programs leading to master's and doctoral degrees in nursing. The common core of knowledge and skills is derived from the conceptual framework that is the structure of the discipline.

## USE OF A CONCEPTUAL FRAMEWORK

The same framework was used in Chapters 5 and 6 to demonstrate a conceptually-based curriculum for baccalaureate and associate degree programs. This was done purposefully to use the structure of the discipline as one approach to facilitate articulation between programs. The program objectives, course titles, and course objectives presented in those chapters are repeated here to compare similarities and differences.

### PROGRAM OBJECTIVES

| ASSOCIATE DEGREE PROGRAM | BACCALAUREATE DEGREE PROGRAM |
|---|---|
| 1. Implement nursing care for individuals and groups who are under the supervision of a professional nurse. | 1. Integrate knowledge of human–environment interactions to promote health, maintain health, regain health, and prevent illness in planning, implementing, and evaluating nursing care of individuals and groups. |
| 2. Use nursing actions to help individuals who are ill return to a functional state of health. | 2. Interpret the interrelationship of perceptions, communications, and transactions, in human interactions of nurses, clients, families, and health professionals in helping individuals who are ill return to health. |
| 3. Support the ethical values of professional nursing | 3. Integrate ethical values of professional nursing in decision making in nursing and health care. |
| 4. Perform functions within secondary health-care systems with the guidance of a professional nurse | 4. Use relevant knowledge from basic sciences, behavioral sciences, humanities, and nursing in planning, implementing, and evaluating effectiveness of nursing care for individuals and groups in primary, secondary, |

5. Appraise effectiveness of technical aspects of nursing care.

6. Participate as a member of the nursing team to deliver care for individuals and groups.

7. Skill in performing observations, measurements, and techniques of nursing with accuracy.

8. Participate in continuing education to add to knowledge and to increase skills.

and tertiary health-care systems.

5. Demonstrate responsibility and accountability for nursing care of individuals and groups.

6. Interpret the independent collaborative functions of professional nurses.

7. Use a theory of goal attainment for professional nursing in working with individuals and groups to facilitate optimum health to function in usual social roles.

8. Demonstrate mastery in performance of basic and advanced technical skills.

9. Formulate a life plan for continuing personal and professional development.

The objectives are listed side by side for ease in comparing similarities and differences in expectations of graduates of each of the programs.

The behavioral terms are at different levels in the taxonomies of educational objectives. In the associate degree program, the behaviors range from knowledge to evaluation, but the content is limited. In the baccalaureate degree program, the behaviors in the objectives tend to be at the level of analysis, synthesis, and evaluation. The similarities are also explicit. For example, the baccalaureate degree graduate is expected to integrate ethical values of professional nursing in decision making in nursing and health care, whereas the associate degree graduate is expected to be aware of and to support the Code for Nurses.

The use of theoretical concepts and application of theoretical knowledge in implementation and evaluation of nursing and health care can be seen in the stated objectives in the baccalaureate program. This provides for increased knowledge of substantive content reflected in the concepts developed by learners. In the associate degree program objectives, the learners develop similar concepts at a basic level of knowledge for use in a structured work situation. The associate degree graduates are integral members of the nursing team, whereas the baccalaureate degree graduates are expected to function independently in the professional role and collaboratively with members of the health team. Within each of these programs, the objectives guide faculty members in selecting learning activities that socialize students into the role for which they are being prepared. Another similarity is in the expectation that graduates from the two programs will continue their education to keep themselves updated in knowledge and skills.

**Courses.** There are similarities and differences in the titles of the courses in the curricula. Requirements for admission to the nursing major vary from one program to another. Some programs plan for students to enroll in nursing courses at the freshman or sophomore level. Other programs begin with one or two nursing courses in the freshman and sophomore years, with emphasis on liberal arts and science, and then decrease the arts and science courses in the junior and senior years and increase the nursing courses. One way to organize a curriculum to facilitate articulation is the completion of all or most of the basic and behavioral sciences and the humanities courses prior to enrolling in the nursing courses in the junior and senior years.

In most instances in the associate degree program, students are admitted and take courses concurrently with the nursing courses. There may be some variations but not many. In the baccalaureate program, the courses must be selected from the various disciplines of the basic and behavioral sciences and the humanities. In the associate degree program, courses may be selected from the basic and behavioral sciences and the humanities that are considered "transfer" courses, or they may take courses called "general education," which are designed for "terminal" programs.

The nursing titles are listed to show some differences, although such a comparison can only be done objectively by analyzing the course objectives, content, learning activities, teaching strategies, and evaluation.

## COURSE TITLES

| ASSOCIATE DEGREE | BACCALAUREATE DEGREE |
|---|---|
| Introduction to Nursing | Historical and Philosophical Foundations of Nursing |
| Practicum in Introduction to Nursing | Theories of Nursing |
| Nursing Skills Laboratory | Introduction to Nursing: Concepts, Process, and Skills |
| | Practicum in Introduction to Nursing |
| | Basic Skills Laboratory |
| Nursing of Individuals | Principles of Teaching and Learning |
| Practicum in Nursing of Individuals | Nursing in Community |
| | Practicum in Community Nursing |
| | Ethical and Legal Dimensions of Nursing |
| Nursing of Groups of Individuals | Nursing in Groups |
| Practicum in Nursing of Groups of Individuals | Practicum in Nursing in Groups |
| Skills Laboratory | Nursing of Individuals |
| | Practicum in Nursing of Individuals |
| | Advanced Skills Laboratory |
| Role and Functions in Technical Nursing | Role and Functions of Professional Nurse |
| Practicum in Functioning in Role of Technical Nurse | Practicum in Functioning in Role of Professional Nurse |
| Issues and Trends in Nursing | Electives in Nursing and other Disciplines |

One similarity in the final semester of each program is that experiences are offered for students to function in the role for which they are being prepared. Another is that skills are an essential component in each of the programs. Also, students learn about nursing care of individuals as individuals and also individuals as members of groups.

One more comparison will be made to show how a conceptual framework based on the structure of the subject of a discipline such as nursing can be used to develop curricula that provide for articulation between ADN and BSN programs.

**Course Objectives.** The objectives for the course titled Introduction to Nursing in the associate degree program and the course titled Introduction to Nursing: Concepts, Process, and Skills in the baccalaureate degree program are compared.

ASSOCIATE DEGREE

1. Outline a general systems framework for the curriculum.

2. Distinguish between facts and inferences in gathering data from observations and measurements of clients' health status.

3. Identify the dependency of a client from each age group in performing activities of daily living.

4. Describe differences in the perceptions of an adolescent and an older adult about health practices.

5. Demonstrate health practices in activities of daily living.

6. Demonstrate skills in basic nursing techniques related to activities of daily living.

7. Demonstrate use of an objective tool to gather information about clients' health status.

BACCALAUREATE DEGREE

1. Discuss a general systems framework for nursing and a theory of goal attainment.

2. Demonstrate communication, both verbal and nonverbal, in gathering reliable information through participant and nonparticipant observations of individuals of all age groups.

3. Identify the dependency of a patient/client from each age group in performing activities of daily living.

4. Verify accuracy of one's perceptions of patient/client status with patient/client perception of his/her health status.

5. Demonstrate skill in health assessment of individuals in each age group.

6. Identify at least five common psychosocial variables in nurse/patient and nurse/family interactions.

7. Describe similarities and differences in health-care agencies in which nurses function.

From the comparisons presented here, one can see similarities and differences in the curricula. When faculty members discuss the differences in general and abstract terms such as depth and breadth, the similarities and differences are unclear. When a side by side comparison is presented, however, the approach to curriculum development and instruction in the two programs is clarified.

Individuals who consider themselves experts in curriculum development and instruction in nursing may have a different approach to demonstrate concrete and specific similarities and differences in associate degree and baccalaureate degree programs. However, use of the same conceptual framework to develop the curricula will facilitate articulation of graduates from the ADN to the BSN program by identification of the entrance behaviors expected and by diagnostic and summative evaluation of the learners to give advanced standing at the junior or senior level.

## A SECOND POINT OF VIEW

Some nurse educators reject the idea that articulation from ADN to BSN is possible. Articulation is not the same as the ladder concept. The latter implies that one must step on one rung of the ladder first before stepping on the second rung. This concept indicates that the ADN is the basic program in nursing preceding the BSN. These are two different programs and one is not basic to the other program. The purposes for these two programs have been clouded over in the past decade because of changes in curricula in ADN programs in which a leadership and management component has been added. There is a need to clarify the real differences philosophically and then to build curricula to reflect the real differences. The myth that one is better than the other must also be dispelled. Each program has a different purpose which should be reflected in the curricula. How can one compare two programs with different purposes and goals?

Articulation as defined here means that the programs are distinct but can be joined by intelligent planning in developing curricula. For those nurse educators who disagree with articulation and to others who disagree with the system of nursing education, some questions are asked for their discussion, debate, and research in determining appropriate educational programs for professional nursing for the future.

## Questions for Discussion

One approach that may help to solve the problem of articulation from ADN to BSN during this transition period in nursing education (BSN is required for entry into the profession) has been presented. Several questions must be discussed, debated, and answered by nurse educators in the near future. A major problem in this educational controversy persists.

How can nurse educators continue to support the BSN as the first professional degree when other professions prepare individuals in post-baccalaureate programs? With the continuous explosion of knowledge in sciences, how can nurse educators continue to implement curricula that do not provide the knowledge required of professional nurses to function in the complex technological world of the health-care systems as equal partners with other professionals? How can nurse educators continue to delete the humanities, especially philosophy, logic, language, English, history, and fine arts, and require only professionally related courses?

In this age of science and technology, a personal and human approach to health care must be maintained. Nursing is the profession that has consistently coordinated health care, which makes it imperative that some semblance of liberal education be maintained in the curricula. Some nurse educators may respond by saying, "Well, if we continue to add more science and mathematics we have to delete something." Maybe this is the reason a BSN is not the decision for the future education for professional nursing. Maybe entry-level education must go beyond undergraduate preparation. These ideas are reported here because that is what a few nurse educators have discussed during the past few years. What research data was made available in the small committee of the American Nurses Association that presented this decision on entry into practice? Data were presented, for example, about the health needs of society, the nutritional needs of society as a basis for healthy people, current disease statistics, and chronic health problems. What knowledge and skills are essential for nurses to function as professionals in the health-care system? Where is the research to accompany major decisions for the future of nursing education? Associate degree programs were initiated on the basis of a five-year study. Where is the research to indicate the basis for BSN programs?

Analogies are often made in comparing nursing to other professions. Sociologists have constantly studied nursing as a profession, and most have stated it is "evolving," "new," or a semi-profession. Another series of questions are asked.

Do you know of any curricula in higher education in which programs for dental assistants articulate with dental hygienists? Do you know of any programs for dental hygienists that articulate with the preparation of dentists? If not, why insist on this in nursing?

Do you know of any curricula for physician's assistants that articulate with programs that prepare physicians? Do you know of curricula for pharmacy technicians that articulate with the programs that train pharmacists? Ask these same questions of any professional curriculum. If other professions prepare individuals for entry into a profession at the post-baccalaureate level, why do nurses and nurse educators continue this pattern? Could one of the reasons be that a national research and development project to determine appropriate curricula to prepare professional nurses for tomorrow has not been conducted? Has the basic problem in nursing education been identified?

This writer has tried to present two sides to a controversy in nursing education. For the present time in nursing education, the problem of articulation should have some attention when faculty groups decide to revise current curricula to provide a way for nurses to meet the educational qualifications of a BSN for the future.

## Articulation between BSN and Graduate Study

Using your imagination, the same curriculum concepts can be used to plan articulation from the baccalaureate degree program to a master's degree program and on through the doctoral degree program in nursing. This is the decade in which nursing educators can demonstrate leadership in curriculum development and instruction in higher education. This type of articulation is one approach to building the discipline of nursing in higher education.

The curriculum guidelines presented in previous chapters can serve a useful purpose for faculty engaged in curriculum development and instruction for new programs. These same concepts can be useful for faculty members engaged in evaluation of current curricula with a plan for revision for the future of nursing as a discipline. From practical experiences in developing curricula in nursing in higher education and years of curriculum consultation with faculty groups, some observation notes on curriculum revision are presented in the next chapter.

# chapter
# 8

# Notes
# on Curriculum
# Revision

The previous chapters discussed approaches for curriculum development and instruction. These ideas are useful in curriculum revision. However, while curriculum changes are planned by faculty members, they must simultaneously preserve the integrity of the current curriculum and provide appropriate learning experiences for students. This twofold direction requires additional faculty expenditure of energy and time to maintain quality in the ongoing curriculum and work on revisions.

Fatigue and frustration may occur in the faculty group. A major problem that tends to occur in curriculum group work is resistance to change. Guidelines for prevention or solution of this and other potential problems are presented. An assumption is made that different leaders in the faculty group will emerge at different times, depending on the tasks and the goals to be achieved. However, to maintain some organization and coordinate the project, an elected or appointed leader will facilitate the work of the group. Organizing for planned change and a rationale for curriculum revision are presented.

## ORGANIZING FOR PLANNED CURRICULUM CHANGE

Curriculum revision requires open communication and purposeful interactions among faculty members and among faculty, students, administrators, individuals, and groups in the community. A clear definition of the goals to be achieved provides criteria for organizing and planning for change.

Curriculum change involves a wide range of human relations. Key concepts in planning and implementing change are communication and purposeful interactions. The following guidelines are offered for organizing for the change process to be implemented.

**1. Active participation in identifying problems, establishing goals, and the means to attain them, will set a climate that is free and flexible.**

Group identification of its own problems can sometimes be a difficult process. If new faculty members are part of the group, they may be able to offer ideas about problems as they perceive them and may be somewhat more detached from past curriculum experiences. Tact is often necessary to prevent adverse reactions to new ideas. One approach to get the group to identify problems is to have the members discuss their ideas about areas they believe should be changed. Some members of the group may introduce several research studies in learning, teaching, and curriculum change. The group leader should bring to the meeting some summaries of the evaluations of the current curriculum. These evaluations would include the students' evaluation of courses and teachers, faculty members' course evaluations, total program evaluations, and evaluations from health-care agencies in which the graduates are employed. Another source of information, the explosion of knowledge from nursing research and changing factors in the health-care systems, would be helpful for discussion.

**2. Mutual respect for the knowledge and experience each faculty member communicates to the group is essential in planning for change.**

One of the barriers to communication in a group, and hence to understanding, is that individuals tend to make judgments about ideas and persons without ever really hearing what is said. One of the ways to break this barrier in group work is to listen to the ideas of others and to ask questions until some understanding is reached. Mutual respect stems from each individual's philosophy of life and from the democratic principle that each human being has worth.

Another barrier in group work may be the fact that some faculty members have had little knowledge or experience in working in task-oriented groups. If this is true for the majority, it may be prudent to have several sessions in group training and in listening before beginning the change process.

**3. Bringing about change in a curriculum may require change in attitudes, and this depends upon the degree to which the individuals are involved in the change process.**

Once the decision has been made to revise the curriculum, those faculty members who will be responsible for implementing the change should be directly involved in the process. Usually the curriculum leader has a responsibility for maintaining enthusiasm in the group and helping members focus on the goals they have defined.

**4. Genuine change will take place when new knowledge, skills, values, and attitudes are perceived by individuals.**

This is an expected outcome of active participation by all faculty members who will be responsible for implementing the changes. Too often in the past, changes were made by a few, and the new curriculum was merely a paper change rather than a genuine change. Some faculty members who have had little or no knowledge from the profession of education remark that total curriculum revision is a waste of time. Their belief is that if they can practice nursing, they can teach it. On the other hand, those faculty members who have knowledge from education can demonstrate that it takes more than being an expert practitioner to be able to teach someone to become a professional nurse. One can argue, too, that those who have knowledge about teaching and learning cannot teach that which they cannot practice. This type of philosophical disagreement within faculty groups engaged in curriculum revision must be resolved if change is to take place.

**5. To arrive at a satisfactory means to a common goal of quality nursing education requires involvement of all faculty and coordination of efforts of all individuals.**

This guideline calls for mutual agreement about the goals to be achieved, the time factor involved in the process, and the selection of one person to coordinate the work of the group

For unity and cohesion to occur in a diversified faculty group, the person selected to coordinate the work of the group should be skilled in communications, interactions, and coordination. A climate that is free and open for dialogue and permits some flexibility within the structure and goals of the group will facilitate effective group work.

**6. The type of administration and its effects on the work structure of the institution from the standpoint of authority, power, status, subgroups, and communication may be factors in faculty resistance to curriculum change.**

Some understanding of the administrative and organizational structure of the college or university is essential for functioning as a responsible and accountable faculty member. Horizontal and vertical communications, informal and formal, are necessary to resolve disparate views, vested interests in a specialty area of nursing, or conflict within the group. Communications and interactions are key factors in moving the group toward the achievement of goals, and often help bring about conflict resolution. Forces of interference may prevent the group from moving forward. For example, if the group is presented with too many new ideas at one time, it may not be able to cope with them; if any member has had a negative experience in faculty curriculum change in the past, that person may be very cautious or passive in the group. One approach is to begin with something the faculty members have in common and move to those ideas that are new and different.

**8. A sense of integrity and ordinary honesty in relations with colleagues will build and maintain the morale of the group.**

Sometimes integrity is lost in today's busy world. Ordinary honesty with colleagues is basic to establishing relationships in a group. Courage is another quality that emerges in a group when a member is seen voting as a minority of one because of a personal principle. In some instances, the facts speak for themselves and decisions are easy to make in the group. One approach may be to gather as many facts about a problem as possible, review the choices and the consequences of each choice, and try to make as rational a decision as possible for that specific situation and time. Remember, decisions can be changed and should be changed when new ideas and new information are available. Patience, tolerance, and understanding are essential qualities for curriculum development and revision.

**9. Administrative support in the allocation of time and material resources for faculty to be able to achieve the goals is absolutely essential.**

In some situations, a grant to secure external funds to engage in curriculum revision is a requirement of a college. Faculty members should be given some time to write grants for funding.

## RATIONALE FOR CURRICULUM REVISION

The role of the curriculum leader is clarified at the beginning of the project. The goals to be achieved and the time to do so are clearly defined by the group. The tasks to accomplish the goals are identified and subgroups formed to work on the tasks and present to the group for review and decisions.

The following areas are to be considered by the total faculty:

1. A decision based on evaluation data is made about the overall aim of the new curriculum.

2. Subgroups are formed to work on specific elements, such as a philosophy group, a conceptual framework group, and a program objectives group.

3. Working papers are distributed from the work of the subgroups to all faculty for review, suggestions, additions, deletions, and questions.

4. Large group meetings are held to make decisions.

5. After agreement is reached about the philosophy for the curriculum and the conceptual framework, program objectives are discussed and agreed upon as working

objectives. Keep in mind that using this approach of working papers and decisions on tentative agreement is essential for the group to move forward. At least one faculty member in every group has an ability to conceptualize the materials of the group and to analyze the total work as a system. That individual can be assigned to look at the working documents for continuity, balance, consistency, adequacy, sequence, etc., and offer suggestions throughout the process for clarification of different components of the curriculum. The idea is that all components should flow one from another and spiral back on the other.

6. After there is faculty agreement on the working philosophy, the conceptual framework, and program objectives, small groups may be formed to identify the courses that will be prerequisite and the courses that will be required for the nursing major.

7. After courses are identified and organized into the educational system either by quarters or semesters, subgroups are formed to design each course, which includes objectives, prerequisites, diagnostic evaluation for determining entry behaviors, content, learning activities, teaching strategies, and formative and summative evaluation.

8. When the courses are completed, faculty members meet as a total group and review the total curriculum. At this time suggestions for refinement of objectives and other components are completed.

9. When the new curriculum has been approved by appropriate committees or councils within the college and university, approval by a board of trustees may be required before faculty initiate plans for implementation and continuous evaluation.

The process of curriculum revision can be an exciting and intellectually stimulating experience for faculty members. Requisites for curriculum revision, implementation, and evaluation are: clearly defined goals and tasks; clearly defined roles and functions of faculty, students, administrators, and community representatives; adequate resources; and time.

The details for curriculum development and diagrams that were discussed in Chapters 5 and 6 are useful in curriculum revisions. The same curriculum and instruction process used for developing a curriculum will facilitate faculty organization in planning for revisions. Prior to this planning, evaluation data from several sources should have been collected for review by the faculty about the kind of changes suggested in the evaluations. This information is added to faculty ideas about the need for changes, the trends in the profession, the explosion of knowledge from nursing research, and the new technologies in health-care systems. The curriculum revision process is shown in Figure 8.1.

When decisions are made to revise a curriculum in a college or a university, information must be gathered to document the need for a revision. The information has usually been collected on a continuous basis in accredited programs. For example, information is collected systematically from the graduates who evaluate the program. Continuous evaluation data is collected from students in the program as they evaluate the courses, learning activities, and evaluation process. A systematic plan for gathering evaluation data about the performance of graduates from the employers in the community provides valuable information. Data about the achievement of graduates on the state licensing examination is helpful. Data about the student population admitted and graduated from the program is available. You may have other kinds of information that would be helpful in making decisions for curriculum revision.

Subsequent to analyzing the evaluation data, a decision may be made to engage in a complete curriculum revision. The process used in Chapters 5 and 6 to develop curricula is useful and is shown again in Figure 8.2.

A suggestion is offered that facilitates implementation of a revised curriculum. Evaluation of the implementation process is essential information for faculty. Once again reference is made

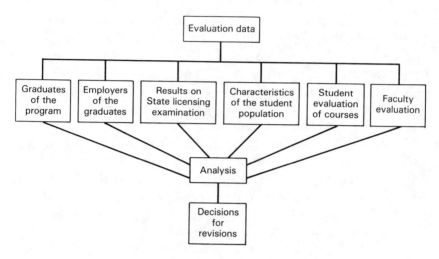

**Figure  8.1**
Curriculum Revision Process

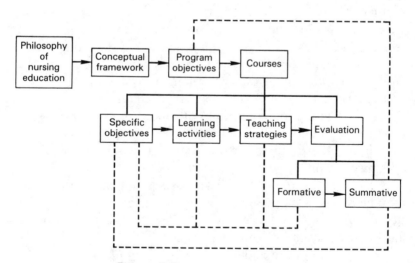

**Figure  8.2**
Curriculum and Instruction Process

to the CIPP model, which provides for continuous evaluation for decision making in developing and implementing a curriculum (Stufflebeam, 1971). Steele (1978) provided a detailed use of this model in nursing.

The "new look" in curriculum development in nursing proposes using the structure of the subject called nursing as the organizing focus. In addition, teaching the student to distinguish between content and process is important. Process provides learning experiences for students to engage in analytical modes of thinking so the students see the relationship between process and content. Strategies for teaching intellectual skills of inductive and deductive reasoning, critical analysis, and scientific inquiry must be learned by teachers so these experiences can be thoroughly integrated into all courses. If there is to be a difference between education for professional nursing and for technical nursing, one difference would be the linking of concepts, skills, and values through the use of an intellectual process as part of every experience. A thumbnail sketch of the future curriculum for the discipline of nursing from the baccalaureate through the doctorate is presented in the final chapter.

## REFERENCES FOR PART II

American Nurses Association. "First Position on Education for Nursing." *American Journal of Nursing* 65, 123 (1965): 106–11.

American Nurses Association. *Standards for Nursing Practice.* Kansas City, Mo.: American Nurses Association, 1973.

American Nurses Association. *Code for Nurses with Interpretive Statements.* Kansas City, Mo.: American Nurses Association, 1976.

American Nurses Association. "Identification and Titling of Establishment of Two Categories of Nursing Practice." *American Nurse,* 1978.

Benson, P.A. "Have we lost sight of the AD philosophy?" *Nursing Outlook* 24 (1977):511–13.

Bloom, B.S., ed. *Taxonomy of Educational Objectives: Cognitive Domain.* New York: Longmans, Green and Co., 1956.

Bloom, B.S.; Hastings, J.T.; and Madaus, G.F. *Handbook on Formative and Summative Evaluation of Student Learning.* New York: McGraw-Hill, 1971.

Bloom, B.S. *et al. Mastery Learning: Theory and Practice.* New York: Holt, Rinehart and Winston, 1971.

Bloom, B.S.; Madaus, G.F.; and Hastings, J.T. *Evaluation to Improve Learning.* New York: McGraw-Hill, 1981.

Bloom, M., and Fischer, J. *Evaluating Practice: Guidelines for the Accountable Professional.* Englewood Cliffs, N.J.: Prentice-Hall, 1982.

Brown, E.L. *Nursing for the Future.* New York: Russell Sage Foundation, 1948.

Bruner, J.S. *The Process of Education.* New York: Vantage Books, 1960.

Carroll, J.B. "A model of school learning." *Teachers College Record* 64 (1963):723–33.

Chapman, J.J. "Microteaching: How students learn group patient education skills." *Nurse Educator* III, 2 (1976):13–16.

Davidson, L., and Knopf, L. *The Community College and Associate Degree Nursing.* New York: National League for Nursing, 1979.

Davis, B.G. "Clinical Expertise as a Function of Educational Preparation." *Nursing Research* 21 (1972):530–34.

Davis, B.G. "Effect of Levels of Nursing Education on Patient Care: A Replication." *Nursing Research* 23 (1974):150–55.

DeChow, H. *Curriculum Design for Associate Degree Nursing Programs.* New York: National League for Nursing, 1978.

Eggen, P.D.; Kauchak, D.P.; and Harder R.J. *Strategies for Teachers*. Englewood Cliffs, N.J.: Prentice-Hall, 1979.

Fawcett, J. *Analysis and Evaluation of Conceptual Models of Nursing*. Philadelphia: F.A. Davis, 1984.

Fraenkel, J.R. *How to Teach About Values: An Analytic Approach*. Englewood Cliffs, N.J.: Prentice-Hall, 1977.

Goldstein, J.O. "Comparison of Graduating ADN and Baccalaureate Nursing Students' Characteristics." *Nursing Research* 29 (1980):46–48.

Gray, J.E.; Murray, B.L.; Roy, J.F.; and Sawyer, J.R. "Do Graduates of Technical and Professional Nursing Programs Differ in Practice?" *Nursing Research* 26 (1977):368–73.

Green, J.L., and Stone, J.C. *Curriculum Evaluation Theory and Practice*. New York: Springer, 1977.

Gronlund, N.E. *Constructing Achievement Tests*. 3rd ed. Englewood Cliffs, N.J.: Prentice-Hall, 1982.

Howell, F.J. "Employers' Evaluations of New Graduates." *Nursing Outlook* 26 (1978):448–436.

Huckabay, L.M. *Conditions of Learning and Instruction in Nursing*. St. Louis, Mo.: C.V. Mosby, 1980.

Inhelder, B., and Piaget, J. *The Early Growth of Logic in the Child*. New York: W.W. Norton, 1964.

King, I.M. *Toward a Theory for Nursing*. New York: John Wiley & Sons, 1971.

King, I.M. "A Process for Developing Concepts for Nursing Through Research." In *Nursing Research I*, edited by P.J. Verhonick. Boston: Little, Brown and Company, 1975.

King, I.M. "The Decision-Maker's Perspective: Patient Aspects." In *Operations Research in Health Care*, edited by L.J. Sharman, R.D. Speas, and J.P. Young. Baltimore: Johns Hopkins University Press, 1975.

King, I.M. "The Health Care System: Nursing Intervention Subsystem." In *Health Research: The Systems Approach*, edited by H.H. Werley, A. Zuzich, M. Zajkowski, and A.D. Zagornik. New York: Springer, 1976.

King, I.M. "How Does the Conceptual Framework Provide Structure for the Curriculum?" In *Curriculum Process for Developing or Revising a Baccalaureate Nursing Program*. New York: National League for Nursing, 1978.

King, I.M. "Notes on Philosophy of Nursing Education." Unpublished, 1980.

King, I.M. *A Theory for Nursing: Concepts, Process, Systems*. New York: John Wiley & Sons, 1981.

King, I.M. "King's Theory of Nursing. Part III." In *Family Health: A Theoretical Approach to Nursing Care*, edited by I.W. Clements, and F.W. Roberts. New York: John Wiley & Sons, 1983.

King, I.M. "National Survey of Philosophies of Nursing Education." *Western Journal of Nursing Research* 6, (1984): 387–404.

Krathwohl, D.R.; Bloom, B.S.; and Masia, B.R. *Taxonomy of Educational Objectives: Affective Domain*. New York: David McKay, 1964.

Lenburg, C. "External Degree in Nursing: The Promise Fulfilled." *Nursing Outlook* 24 (1976):422–29.

Lenburg, C. *The Clinical Performance Examination*. New York: Appleton-Century-Crofts, 1979.

Mager, R.F. *Preparing Instructional Objectives*. Palo Alto, Ca.: Fearon Publishers, 1962.

Meisenhelder, J.B. "Clinical Evaluation-An Instructor's Dilemma." *Nursing Outlook* 30 (1982):348–51.

Montag, M. *Community College Education for Nursing*. New York: McGraw-Hill, 1959.

Montag, M. *The Education of Nurse Technicians.* New York: G.P. Putnam's Sons, 1951.

National League for Nursing. *Characteristics of Associate Degree Education in Nursing.* Pub. No. 23-1500. New York: National League for Nursing, 1973.

National League for Nursing. *Characteristics of Baccalaureate Programs in Nursing.* New York: National League for Nursing, 1978.

National League for Nursing. *Competencies of the Associate Degree Nurse on Entry into Practice.* Pub. No. 23-1731. New York: National League for Nursing, 1978.

National League for Nursing Education. *Characteristics of Associate Degree Nursing Programs.* New York: NLNE, 1960.

Nelson, L.F. "Competence of Nursing Graduates in Technical, Communicative, and Administrative Skills." *Nursing Research* 27 (1978):121-25.

Palmer, P.E., and Brown, S.K. "AD Challenge Exams: Two Approaches." *Nursing Outlook* 22 (1974): 584-86.

Partridge, K.B. "Nursing Values in a Changing Society." *Nursing Outlook* 26 (1978):356-60.

Peterson, C.J.; Broderick, M.E.; Demarest, L.; and Holey L. *Competency-Based Curriculum and Instruction.* New York: National League for Nursing, 1979.

Popham, W.J. *Criterion-Referenced Measurement.* Englewood Cliffs, N.J.: Prentice-Hall, 1978.

Popham, W.J. *Modern Educational Measurement.* Englewood Cliffs, N.J.: Prentice-Hall, 1981.

Reilly, D.E. *Behavioral Objectives: Evaluation in Nursing.* 2nd ed. New York: Appleton-Century-Crofts, 1980.

Rogers, C.R. *Freedom to Learn.* Columbus, Oh.: Charles Merrill, 1969.

Schwirian, P.M. "Evaluating the Performance of Nurses: A Multi-Dimensional Approach." *Nursing Research* 27 (1978):347–51.

Simpson, E.J. *The Classification of Educational Objectives: Psychomotor Domain*. Urbana, Ill.: University of Illinois Press, 1966.

Snyder, J.C., and Wilson, M.F. "Elements of a Psychological Assessment." *American Journal of Nursing* 77 (1977): 235–41.

Sommerfeld, D.P., and Accola, K.M. "Evaluating Students' Performance." *Nursing Outlook* 26 (1978):432–36.

Steele, S. *Educational Evaluation in Nursing*. Thorofare, N.J.: Charles B. Slack, 1978.

Stufflebeam, D.L., ed. *Educational Evaluation and Decision Making*. Itaska, Ill.: F.E. Peacock, 1971.

Thorndike, R.L., and Hagen, E. *Measurement and Evaluation in Psychology and Education*. 3rd ed. New York: John Wiley & Sons, 1969.

Tier, L.L., and DeAngelis, B.R. *Curriculum Design for Associate Degree Nursing Programs: Teaching and Evaluation in the Classroom*. New York: National League for Nursing, 1980.

Torres, G., and Yura, H. *Today's Conceptual Framework: Its Relationship to the Curriculum Development Process*. New York: National League for Nursing, 1974.

Tuttle, H.S. "A Wholesome Philosophy Misapplied." *Educational Forum* 27, 3 (1963):289–95.

Tyler, R. *Curriculum and Instruction*. Chicago: University of Chicago Press, 1949.

Waltz, C.E., Strickland, O.L., Lenz, R.R., *Measurements in Nursing Research*. Philadelphia: F.H. Davis, 1984.

Waters, V.H.; Vivier, M.L.; Chater, S.S.; Urrea, J.J.; and Wilson, H.S. "Technical and Professional Nursing: An Exploratory Study." *Nursing Research* 21 (1972):124–30.

Waters, V.H. *Distinguishing Characteristics of Associate Degree Education For Nursing.* New York: National League for Nursing, 1978.

Whitehead, A. *Adventures in Ideas.* New York: Pelican Books, 1948.

Wilson, N.L. *Curriculum Design for Associate Degree Nursing Programs. Two Challenges: Implementing a Conceptual Framework and Pre- and Post-Clinical Conferences.* New York: National League for Nursing, 1980.

Wolf, V.C., and Quiring, J. "Carroll's Model Applied to Nursing Education." *Nursing Outlook* 19 (1971):176–79.

Yura, H. and Walsh, M. *The Nursing Process.* New York: Appleton-Century-Crofts, 1983.

# *chapter* 9
# Nursing Curricula for the Future

## INTRODUCTION

The last part of this book presents ideas for educators and researchers to discuss as they develop educational nursing programs in higher education. Future curricula for the education of individuals for professional nursing should reflect the structure of the discipline. The discipline is based on a body of knowledge that continues to be identified in theories and in nursing research. The past fifteen years has shown an increase in research in nursing practice. Recently, the need for continuous research in curriculum and instruction has been demonstrated, and a new organization that will focus on this kind of research has been formed. Annual meetings have been held since 1983 to disseminate research findings in nursing education.

In Chapter 9, three areas that focus on nursing as a discipline are explored. First, highlights of studies of nursing education are identified. Second, the fact that nursing meets a social need is shown in measuring nursing as a profession. Nursing meets the criteria by which a profession is evaluated in the United States. Third, nursing is measured against the functions of a discipline, described by Parker and Rubin (1966).

Nursing is an emerging discipline in higher education. Nurse educators are urged to continue to evaluate curricula and make revisions in undergraduate programs leading to a baccalaureate degree with a major in nursing. The revisions would include a study of conceptual systems for nursing, theories for nursing, intellectual and scientific skills, and the basic and advanced skills of a clinician. These areas of content serve as a foundation for a discipline, which is introduced to students in the undergraduate program in accepted academic disciplines. A hypothetical curriculum is suggested for discussing, thinking about, and considering curricula revisions in undergraduate and graduate programs to indicate the structure of the subject called nursing.

The last chapter of the book suggests the importance of a cadre of nurses who will continue to conduct research in nursing and nursing education. One area of relevance is agreement as a profession on the domain for professional nursing, to establish boundaries within which research problems can be studied and methods to solve them can be identified. Another area of relevance is the need to select concepts that have occurred in the nursing literature over the years and perceived by nurses as basic content and as essential knowledge for the practice of professional nursing. These common concepts should be subjected to objective study to determine construct validity.

## NURSING—AN INTELLECTUAL DISCIPLINE

Several elements have been identified that are essential for naming a field of study an intellectual discipline. Initially, science tends to look for patterns of relations to describe natural phenomena of interest in a field of study. Patterns are organized in discovering sets of concepts in a relationship, designing conceptual frameworks, or constructing theories. These organizing foci, which direct inquiry into relevant questions, define the conceptual component of the structure of a discipline. The syntactical structure of a discipline relates to the methods for using the concepts to achieve goals (Schwab, 1962).

The structure of the subject provides the basis for designing curricula for disciplines in higher education. Nurse educators must begin to think of the discipline of nursing and develop curricula in higher education that reflect the structure of the subject. It is neither efficient nor economical to think of curricula in nursing as separate entities. One of the purposes of this chapter is to suggest a curriculum that may give impetus to thinking about and discussing curriculum revisions to educate professional nurses in the discipline of nursing.

Three major highlights in the history of nursing are discussed prior to suggesting a curriculum for the future of nursing education in the United States. First, selected historical facts about nursing education are reviewed. Second, nursing as a profession is affirmed. Third, nursing as an intellectual discipline in higher education is explored.

## HISTORICAL EVENTS IN NURSING EDUCATION

The period from 1873 to 1893 in the United States was considered a pioneering stage in education, and the history of nursing education is typical of this time. Some nursing schools were established separate from hospitals, according to the pattern of Florence Nightingale, but these were soon modified as evidenced by some of the reports of the U.S. Bureau of Education. Statistics for nursing schools in 1879 were published in the report of the U.S. Commissioner of Education. Eleven schools were established, located predominately in the East, with the exception of the Midwifery School in St. Louis, Missouri. The conditions for admission were based on age, which ranged from twenty-one to forty-five in most schools. A salary of $10.00 per month was paid to the students in the first year, with a $5.00 to $7.00 increase in the second year. The number of students enrolled ranged from six in one school to sixty-four in another school. The length of the program ranged from one to two years (U.S. Commissioner, 1881, pp. 620–621).

Some historians have described the period from 1893 to 1913 as one of phenomenal expansion of schools with little local and professional control (Roberts, 1954). The U.S. Bureau of Education published a report of the educational status of nursing in 1912. This report, written by M. Adelaide Nutting, also described the first course for graduate nurses at Columbia University, Teachers College, New York.

Stress, turmoil, self-examination, and experimentation explained the period from 1913 to 1933. The 1916–18 Biennial Survey of Education recorded data about the phenomenal expansion of hospital schools with some interpretation of the facts. The following quotation from that document is an example:

> Within the past few years the subject of nurse training has received so much attention that it is thought desirable to publish a special chapter on these schools . . . pointing out a number of the most pronounced conditions and tendencies as revealed by the data con-

tained herein. . . . From 1879 to 1893, the number of schools reporting did not exceed one hundred. Since the latter date, the
number of schools has increased from sixty-five to one thousand
seven hundred seventy-six. . . . The rapid growth of schools within
the past five years has been phenomenal. There has been an increase
of forty-two percent in five years. Approximately one hundred new
schools are being organized annually. (Dept. of the Interior, 1921,
pp. 549-646).

Another quotation implies that nursing schools were re-
moved from the status of the profession and from the status of
professional education.

Hitherto, the statistics of nurses training schools have been included with those of theology, law, medicine . . . in the chapter de-
voted to professional education. This year [1918] the statistics of
the other professional schools are included in the chapter on colleges, universities and professional schools, and the statistics of
nurse training schools are printed separately (pp. 549-646).

Facts about nursing education were recorded in the Biennial Surveys of Education in the United States until about 1932.
By 1931, the National League for Nursing Education published
information about nursing schools. A major document for reporting statistics about nursing and nursing education today is
called *Facts About Nursing* (ANA, 1982).

### Nursing Education Studies and Reports

The leaders in nursing history demonstrated a need for
systematic study of nursing and nursing education. One of the
first published reports to guide nursing schools in curriculum
development did not seem to influence changes in programs.
Social sciences were suggested as a part of a nursing curriculum (NLNE, 1917, p. 12). In a second report to assist nursing
schools develop curricula, the functions and responsibilities of
nurses were listed. The case study method was recommended
with an increase in hours spent studying social and health con-

cepts (NLNE, 1927). A third comprehensive guide for curriculum development in schools of nursing was published a decade later (NLNE, 1937). Isabel Stewart, chairperson for the committee, asked many nurses for their opinions. This active participation by nurses resulted in some consensus about a curriculum guide for schools of nursing. Three problems were identified in this report: 1) organization of the curriculum, which included a statement of philosophy, objectives, and standards; 2) selection of learning experiences to help students achieve the objectives; and 3) administration of the curriculum. Optimum standards were discussed and placed within the context of society and its educational system. *A bachelor of science in nursing as a first or basic professional degree was recommended.* The implementation of this recommendation is taking place in several states in 1984.

The first comprehensive study of nursing and nursing education in the United States was published in the 1920's (Goldmark, 1923). This report advocated *two types of practitioners, the professional and practical nurse*, with a need for state registration for both types to protect the public. A need for *financial assistance to develop and strengthen the university school* and to train leaders was indicated.

An eight-year research project, under the auspices of the National League for Nursing Education, was begun in 1926, and the final reports were published by 1934. In one report, the need for radical reform was mentioned.

> The previous studies and reports in nursing have made it clear that there is one fundamental condition that is handicapping progress, a condition which must be removed if satisfactory results were to be achieved. . . . This basic weakness lay in the fact that nursing schools were operated for the most part as adjuncts to the management of hospitals and not primarily as educational institutions (Committee, 1934, p. 23).

This same report indicated the "lack of quality nursing" programs in comparison with other professional schools.

A pamphlet was revised to guide curriculum development,

*Essentials of a Good School of Nursing* (NLNE, 1942). The influence of World War II on society and nursing education is recorded in history books. One event that influenced nursing education was the initiation of the U.S. Cadet Nurse Corps. If schools of nursing wanted to receive tax dollars to increase enrollment and to participate in this program, the curriculum had to be shortened to two-and-a-half years. Students were permitted to select a health-care agency away from the home school for their last six months in the program. At this point in history, most schools were operated by hospitals. Immediately following the war, studies were conducted about nursing education. The Brown report (1948) recommended that education for professional nursing should be planned, implemented, and evaluated by faculty in institutions of higher education. A program leading to *a bachelor of science degree was recommended*.

Following the Brown study, a survey of schools of nursing was conducted and 97 percent of the schools participated. A consistent problem was the lack of understanding as to what constituted education for professional nursing practice. The diversity in curricula in schools and 'the lack of adequately prepared faculty was discussed. Forty-five percent of the nurse faculty members had no academic degree. In addition, these faculty members taught several subjects (West and Hawkins, 1950).

The Ginsberg report (1950) *recommended* that nursing consider *two categories of workers*, the *professional and the practical nurse*. A small volume that called for some action in nursing education recommended the education of nurse technicians (Montag, 1951). This study suggested that the functions of the registered nurse of that period could be taught in a specially designed curriculum and implemented in a community college. In addition, a recommendation was made that the faculty and administrators for these programs have advanced preparation in masters degree programs to function in the role of teacher or administrator.

A five-year research study in which the ideas of Montag were implemented in selected educational institutions in the

United States demonstrated that preparation for functions of the registered nurse can take place in programs leading to an associate degree in community colleges (Montag, 1959).

A report of a survey of collegiate schools of nursing noted the great diversity in collegiate education. Those institutions of higher education offering credit for a baccalaureate degree in nursing were challenged by the nursing organizations in the 1950's.

Two types of baccalaureate curricula were fully approved by the Association of Collegiate Schools of Nursing, the National League for Nursing Education, and the National Nursing Accrediting Service. In one of the types approved by the above organizations, the first two years were spent in academic courses in a college or a university. In the third year, courses were taken in subjects that applied specifically to nursing, such as anatomy. Nursing courses were included in the third year which provided classroom and clinical application under supervision. The fourth and fifth years consisted of a concentration on completing nursing courses.

A second type of program approved by the nursing organizations was organized so that students were enrolled in academic subjects in colleges or universities with one or two basic nursing courses in the first year of a four-year program. The second year was planned so that academic courses decreased in number, courses in related fields applied to nursing were required, and nursing courses increased. In the third year, a few academic courses were required and nursing courses increased. In the first part of the fourth year, academic courses and nursing courses were about the same in number of hours required. The last semester of the fourth year concentrated on nursing courses.

A third type of program was approved if it fulfilled the policies of individual colleges. This program was organized so the majority of courses in the first year were liberal arts and sciences with a few nursing courses. A small part of the second year was spent studying fields related to nursing. The majority of the courses were in nursing. The third year consisted of all nursing courses. About two-thirds of the fourth year consisted of academic courses with a few nursing courses. The last part of the fourth year consisted of nursing courses.

The fourth type of baccalaureate program that existed in the 1950's was not approved by the nursing organizations because institutions of higher education granting the bachelor of science degree were not responsible for the content or level of the courses that comprised the major in nursing. This type of program was called an affiliation between a hospital diploma school and a college or university. Two kinds of affiliations were prevalent. In one type, the students completed a hospital diploma program and enrolled in a college or university for the academic courses and received a bachelor of science degree. In another type of affiliation, students completed two years of academic courses and the last three years were spent in an affiliated hospital school program.

Bridgman's report (1953) discussed in detail and presented graphs of the status of baccalaureate education in nursing in the early 1950's. In this same report, Bridgman noted the role of the junior colleges in providing "terminal-occupational education" in nursing. She mentioned the project by Montag in which selected institutions had begun to implement experimental curricula in two-year programs in selected junior colleges.

A study of nursing education for professional practice was conducted by Lambertson (1958). A clearly stated assumption in this study was that "knowledge, understanding, skills, abilities, attitudes and values essential to nursing team leadership in the hospitals are equally essential to the professional role of nursing in any employment situation or any social setting" (p. 3). Another assumption was made that preparation for nursing team leadership takes place in a collegiate program. The study made a valuable contribution in charting a course for curriculum development for education for professional practice at that period in history. A method for delivery of nursing care, team nursing in hospitals, was an outgrowth of this study.

When the national nursing organizations merged into two organizations, the educational component for nursing was maintained in the newly formed National League for Nursing. Within this new organization, councils for each of four types of pro-grams—baccalaureate, associate, diploma, and practical—were formed. This organization and control of nursing education standards and accreditation policies has been maintained to this day. The accreditation standards provided an organized approach for schools of nursing and at the same time allowed for autonomy and flexibility within each type of program. After the many years of study, some consensus was reached about educational programs for nursing.

The last national survey of nursing and nursing education in the United States was published in 1970 (Lysaught, 1970). The recommendations of previous studies were supported by this report. In addition, one of the first recommendations of the report was to increase the support for research in nursing and nursing education.

One note on the professional organization's responsibility for nursing education is important here. The American Nurses Association Committee on Long Term Goals reported a recommendation to the House of Delegates (ANA, 1960). Goal III of the report stated:

> To insure that, within the next 20-30 years, the education basic to the professional practice of nursing, for those who then enter the profession, shall be secured in a program that provides the intellectual, technical, and cultural components of both a professional and liberal education. Toward this end, the American Nurses Association shall promote the baccalaureate program so that in due course it becomes the basic educational foundation for professional nursing.

In 1965, the ANA position paper on education for the profession for the future was published. In 1978, the House of Delegates of the American Nurses Association passed a resolution. The resolution called for the identification and titling of two categories of nursing practice and for developing a statement of competencies for those categories. By the latter part of 1983, approximately twenty-one state nurses associations were working toward changing laws to implement this decision.

This seems to be an appropriate time to analyze curricula

in higher education for nursing and structure the subject of nursing into an intellectual discipline which will reflect education for professional practice. Can nurse educators learn from the history of nursing? The space age is upon us. Do the curricula in higher education for nursing reflect the knowledge required to function in this age of high technology and the need for continuing humanitarian concern for human beings?

As society increases its technology, specialization in occupations and professions increases. The trend toward specialization in nursing has been the education of clinical specialists in graduate education leading to masters and higher degrees. Another role for which nurses have been prepared has been that of advanced nurse practitioner.

Specific knowledge essential for professional nurses to practice in an age of technology can hardly be taught and learned in a formal four-year education program. Continuing education is a life-long process. There is also a need for continued development of a body of knowledge necessary for the practice of professional nursing.

Within the past ten years, nursing literature has recorded published works that deal with theory development in nursing and research in clinical practice. The debate today is no longer about the question, "Is nursing a profession?"; it is rather about "nursing as an intellectual discipline" in higher education. Before we view nursing as a discipline, we must discuss nursing as a profession.

## NURSING AS A PROFESSION

The criteria commonly used to measure the professional status of a group are summarized to demonstrate that nursing is a profession. The following criteria are adapted from the Bixler's article on the professional status of nursing (Bixler, 1959).

**Criterion 1.** *A profession utilizes an organized body of knowledge to which professionals continuously enlarge the* *body of knowledge through research.* Within the past five years, several nursing research journals have been founded to provide a way to report the increased research in nursing. Analysis of reported studies over the past twenty years shows a change in focus for the studies. Initially, the focus was the study of nurses, roles, and professional organizations. Today, the focus is on studying clinical practice. Recently, the Society for Research in Nursing Education has been formed to provide an avenue for reporting and critiquing research in nursing education. An increased emphasis on theory development and research has been brought about by the increase in numbers of nurses in doctoral programs from 300 in the early 1960's to over 2500 in 1984. A cadre of nurse researchers is essential to continue to add to the body of knowledge. Twenty years ago most nurses earned doctoral degrees in other disciplines. In 1984, at least 22 programs offering doctoral degrees in nursing are admitting students. The nursing profession meets this criterion.

**Criterion 2**. *Education for the profession takes place in institutions of higher education.* Decisions were made by the nursing profession through representation at the American Nurses Association House of Delegates to place nursing education within institutions of higher education (ANA, 1978). Entry into professional practice in the future will require that students complete a baccalaureate program in a college or a university. This decision is being implemented in many states at this time. This criterion has been met in that the majority of nurses are graduating from ADN and BSN programs within higher education in the United States.

**Criterion 3**. *The theoretical knowledge of a profession is used in providing a social service which is deemed vital to human and social welfare in society.* A personal opinion is given that nursing as a profession is progressing more rapidly than other professions in formulating theories for nursing and in testing the ideas in research. In the process of continuing to develop a body of knowledge, nursing has not lost sight of the humanitarian component of the service provided. In fact, some nurses have discussed the fact that values are critical variables in studying natural situations in nursing practice. Theories and research assist nursing to meet this criterion.

**Criterion 4.** *Professionals are autonomous in their functions, control professional standards, promulgate a code of ethics, and make decisions on professional policy.* Evidence of meeting this criterion can be seen in the pronouncements of the American Nurses Association related to national health policy and nursing's responsibility in this arena. A code for nurses has been promulgated by the profession, is reviewed periodically, and changed on the basis of new knowledge and practices. Standards for nursing practice have been published in the major areas of nursing. Nurses function in autonomous roles and also in collaborative roles. They are legally and ethically responsible for their practice. They are accountable to the public they serve and to the profession. This criterion is met.

**Criterion 5.** *Individuals who enter a profession demonstrate commitment to spend their working career within the profession.* Some of the initial health personnel studies demonstrated that nurses remained in the work force as long as and longer than most other occupations in which women were in a majority. In the era of the women's movement in the United States, many more nurses are combining marriage and family with their profession. The increase in men in nursing has been slow but continuous.

**Criterion 6.** *Professionals are compensated through economic security programs and continue to have freedom of action in professional growth.* Although in some areas of nursing the compensation is not based on equal pay for equal worth, changes are forthcoming through a major effort of the American Nurses Association and state nurses' associations. In achieving this criterion, time and energy can be spent in professional growth.

The progress in nursing in the past twenty years has been phenomenal. The age-old argument as to whether or not nursing is a profession must be put to rest so that energy can be spent in identifying theories in nursing and in conducting research to add to the body of knowledge essential for professional practice and for nursing as a discipline.

### Nursing—An Intellectual Discipline

A curriculum movement in the United States in the sixties advocated that all teachers should begin to organize content in their subject matter according to the structure of the disciplines. A report of a conference provided teachers and researchers with ideas about the structure of a discipline and the concept of a spiral curriculum (Bruner, 1960).

A spiral curriculum is one organized to develop concepts at every level of education. For example, elementary school children are assisted to begin to develop a concept of health. This concept can be developed at the secondary school level and again in college and in curricula for health professionals.

The structure of a discipline is a way to organize the content of the subject to be taught in a field of study. Older disciplines such as biology, chemistry, and physiology classified knowledge in a descriptive way. For example, biology identified species, genera, etc.; physiology identified cells, tissues, organs, systems; and chemistry classified elements in a periodic table. The literature in nursing has shown some agreement on what some nurses call a "metaparadigm," consisting of the comprehensive concepts of person, environment, health, and society. The movement in nursing diagnosis for the past decade, describing a classification system for nursing, has shown progress. A variety of ways to organize curricula have been used in nursing, such as body systems, twenty-one problems, a hierarchy of needs, and the medical model. Since the early 1970's, nurse educators have been using a conceptual framework as the organizing focus for curricula.

One of the criteria for evaluating programs for accreditation by the National League for Nursing was the use of a conceptual framework to organize content. At a meeting of the Council of Member Agencies of the Department of Baccalaureate and Higher Degree programs, the term "conceptual framework" was deleted from the criteria (NLN, 1982). Is it possible that conceptual frameworks were constructed for accreditation purposes rather than for the influence they should have on the curriculum? Isn't this decision an interesting one at a time when nursing was beginning to demonstrate structure in the subject? Reference is made to a study in which the analysis of conceptual frameworks in a sample of accredited baccalaureate programs identified major concepts and subconcepts in the programs (Torres & Yura, 1974). The major concepts were man, health, society, and nursing. This kind of information from studies in nursing education will help nurse educators and researchers continue to organize the structure of the subject.

The practice in other disciplines has been to look for patterns of relations among the relevant concepts and for patterns of change. When new patterns are found, they provide new relations from former descriptions of patterns. Many articles and books have been written about the structure of the sciences, the way to become an intellectual discipline, and the differences in conceptual frameworks in nursing (see "References").

Criteria were used to evaluate nursing as a profession. The functions of a discipline suggested by Parker and Rubin (1961) will be used to evaluate nursing as a discipline.

## THE FUNCTIONS OF A DISCIPLINE

### Historical and Philosophical Foundations

The cultural heritage of nursing can be found in its recorded history. When nurse educators deleted a course titled *History of Nursing*, which was taught as a first course in some baccalaureate programs many years ago, they may not have been aware that it was one of the solid academic courses in the curriculum that was recognized and respected by other academicians. The old complaint that this was a boring and dry course reflects on the teachers rather than the substantive content. Christy pointed out so eloquently that nursing in the 1970's and 1980's seems to be repeating itself (Christy, 1980). Without a knowledge of the history of nursing, nurses will continue to repeat the problems of the past. A curriculum for the future should require a course in the history of nursing.

From analysis of recorded history, the philosophical foundations of nursing can be discovered. This writer reviewed the American Journal of Nursing from 1900 to 1960 to identify the definitions of nursing reported for that period. The definitions of nursing reflected the nature of society, the role of women in society, medical practice, the role of nurses, and a concept of health as the goal for nursing. Based on that review of nursing literature, my conceptual framework for nursing indicated that a consistent goal for nursing has been the attainment and maintenance of health for individuals. If people become ill or disabled, nurses help them regain a functional state of health that is individual for each person. If this is not possible, nurses have helped individuals die with dignity (King, 1968, 1971, 1981).

A study of philosophies of nursing education in the United States was conducted (King, 1984). A stratified random sample of philosophies in three different educational programs—diploma, associate degree, and baccalaureate—was selected. Analysis of philosophies indicated differences and commonalities in the terms used. The findings from this study can be generalized, since it was a national survey. Analysis of nursing literature will give nurses some of the philosophical foundations of the profession.

Another area of analysis would be to review and analyze the code for nurses and compare with the nursing literature to find philosophical ideas. Some nurses have identified a concept of holism as a philosophical base for nursing. Existentialism has been discussed the past ten or fifteen years in the literature. Historical research in conjunction with descriptive, quasi-experimental, and experimental research provides a basis for the structure of the discipline.

## Methods of Inquiry

Methods of inquiry in nursing have been influenced by the prevailing philosophy of science over the years. Since doctoral programs in nursing were nonexistent until recently, nurses who wanted research training entered programs in disciplines offering these experiences. They learned the methods of inquiry in a specific discipline, such as sociology, physiology, anthropology, psychology, education, and others.

Recent articles by nurses have indicated that some of the traditional scientific approaches should be reconsidered as they are not always appropriate as methods of inquiry into the nature of nursing (Greene, 1979; Tinkley and Beaton, 1983; Watson, 1981). The conceptual frameworks and theories published by nurses since the early 1970's have been attempts by individuals to outline and define the subject matter of nursing and to direct and control inquiries into the nature of nursing.

## Special Ways of Looking at Phenomena

The findings from research in nursing and the formulation of hypotheses generated by theories have begun to identify special ways of viewing concepts deemed relevant for the discipline, such as stressors in the environment, conservation of energy of individuals, nurse–client interactions, and humanistic and holistic nursing practice. One special way of looking at human beings interacting with environments in nursing studies is called naturalistic inquiry. This special way of studying phenomena takes research out of a laboratory into a natural setting to try to identify some explanatory and predictive knowledge that can be applied in nursing situations to improve care.

**Models for Systematic Thought.**   A recent publication has presented an evaluation of "conceptual models of nursing" (Fawcett, 1984). There are a variety of conceptual frameworks in nursing. Fawcett suggested a framework for analysis and identified some of the commonalities and differences in these nursing frameworks. A commonality in nursing curricula is the use of the "nursing process" as defined and explained by Yura and Walsh (1983). This nursing process is a method for thinking about the process of organizing information to plan, implement, and evaluate nursing care. Research into each element of the process provides interesting information for this nursing process as a model for systematic thought. A model for classification of nurse–patient interactions that lead to transactions in nursing situations is another approach for systematic thought in using a theory of goal attainment in nursing practice, nursing education, and nursing administration (King, 1981, p. 156).

**Accumulation of Information.** A review of nursing literature for at least the past twenty years demonstrates an explosion of information and accumulation of knowledge that is overwhelming in selecting relevant content for nursing curricula. This accumulation of information was a major reason for this writer to conceptualize nursing to cope with the knowledge deemed essential for the practice of professional nursing. Accumulation of information seems to indicate that nurses should begin to validate some of the concepts used in nursing over the years and to organize nursing on the basis of such validation. As information continues to accumulate, new conceptualizations for nursing will be constructed.

**Procedures for Using Research.** Some assumptions are made that nurse educators in graduate programs require that students use research findings to improve nursing practice and nursing education. A few examples are the evaluation of studies about stress in intensive care units in hospitals, stress in hospitalized children and adults, and stress in family relationships, and the organization of the research findings into a useful configuration of knowledge that can be used by graduate students in their practicums.

Another example of a procedure for using research is to provide learning experiences for students to develop relevant concepts from the research literature and formulate a systematic approach for testing the concept in natural nursing situations. A variety of procedures are selected by nurse educators to use research findings. These procedures should be taught in the first course in the nursing major in higher education and experiences sequenced throughout the curriculum.

**Processes for Acquisition of Knowledge.** The nursing process mentioned above serves a very useful purpose for organizing knowledge for nursing. A process of inquiry referred to as an intellectual process helps one acquire knowledge. Concept development is a way of acquiring knowledge. In philosophy of science, processes have been called inductive, deductive, and hypothetico-deductive reasoning. The investigative process for acquiring systematized knowledge has been called the research process.

**Processes for Utilization of Knowledge.** If knowledge is to be utilized, it must be disseminated to nurses. One assumption is made that findings must be shared in a variety of ways before individuals can utilize knowledge. Several mechanisms have been used in nursing over the years to communicate research findings that provide knowledge of the subject of nursing. For example, since 1951 conferences have been held to disseminate research findings in nursing. An increase in the number of research journals has provided more outlets for published results of studies. The growth of chapters of Sigma Theta Tau (the nursing honor society) have shown an increase in annual research conferences to disseminate and critique research findings in nursing.

One problem that continues to exist in nursing is to find a way to help staff nurses in health-care agencies gain new knowledge which may be used in practice. One approach is to require faculty members to keep their knowledge and application to practice updated. In some situations, nurse researchers work collaboratively with staff nurses to design and conduct research relative to problems in the agency. This brings the scientific process and findings close to the place where they can be implemented when relevant to the situation.

**What Unsolved Problems and Questions Confront Nursing?**
Nursing has been concerned with unsolved problems in the delivery of care. Nurses have raised relevant questions that require systematic study of nursing practice in natural situations. These

deal with both the conceptual and syntactical structure of the discipline referred to at the beginning of this chapter. Unsolved problems and questions deal with the identification of relevant concepts and the development and testing of theories that have already been proposed and those that will be proposed in the future. These problems and questions revolve around the interaction of people with the environment which leads to a functional state of health. These concepts of person, environment, and health present unsolved problems and research questions in nursing.

**Learning the Discipline as a System Rather than Facts.** This function of a discipline is one of the problems that nurse educators must confront and solve in the immediate future. If you are a nurse educator, reflect on the courses you are teaching. Are you teaching students facts or are you helping them develop relevant concepts? There is a difference. Teaching for concept development will be more readily visible as nurses continue to delineate the structure of the discipline. The question is, "How do we organize the subject matter of nursing into a system, such as a conceptual framework, so that the relevant concepts, skills, and values in nursing can be learned by students who aspire to become professional nurses?" When nurse educators arrive at a general consensus about the essential concepts, nursing can identify structure for the discipline. We are at the threshold of doing this.

As this writer continues to review the nursing literature, several concepts have become dominant. For example, a concept of caring has received renewed emphasis. The concept of empathy has been studied over the past twenty years. There is accumulated knowledge about stressors and stress. Concepts of movement, time, perception, pain, body rhythms, touch, and others have been studied in nursing. Nurse–client interactions have been studied for years. A concept of interactions is central in a theory of goal attainment in nursing (King, 1981). Nurses must continue to identify those concepts that have appeared consistently in the literature and have been and are being systematically studied.

An attempt to classify nursing is shown in the nursing diagnosis movement. A pronouncement was made at the 1982 national conference that new and currently published nursing diagnosis categories must be based on empirical research. The plea is for more nurses to come to the threshold and help open the doors through critical analysis and thinking, theory development, and research. The results will be knowledge that is useful in delivering an essential service to the public.

The scientific aspects of a discipline go through stages in identifying the domain from which the major subject matter is organized. Several nurses have discussed the discipline of nursing (Donaldson and Crowley, 1978; Greene, 1979; Kim, 1983). Kim noted that "nursing can claim to be a scientific field only by adhering to scientific rules of procedure and this has to be achieved through the development of systematized theoretical statements about relevant questions in nursing" (p. 31). Some scientists view theories as instruments for explaining problems of concern in a discipline. The multiple and diverse conceptual frameworks in nursing have identified problems and raised questions about nursing's domain of investigation.

Using criteria related to the functions of a discipline, nursing meets the criteria in different ways. Modifications are made as new findings from research are disseminated and used. Continuous expansion of the body of knowledge will produce changes in theories. Tentativeness and perpetual movement forward are characteristics of a discipline.

Three major elements in a discipline have been explored. Highlights from studies and reports about the history of education in nursing were reviewed. Examples of problems to be studied in nursing and questions about specific methods of inquiry were noted. The structure of nursing, conceptual and syntactical, was alluded to in its relation to the published conceptual frameworks in nursing and the nurses who are questioning methods of scientific inquiry in nursing. The significance of structure of a discipline is linked to basic human activities. Nursing's development of a body of knowledge is significant for human beings in that the knowledge is used for health promotion, disease prevention, care of persons who are ill and disabled, and care for those who are dying. The health of a community is also a concern of nurses.

Nurse educators have a responsibility to evaluate curricula and to consider revisions that demonstrate that nursing is an intellectual discipline in higher education. A hypothetical curriculum is suggested to stimulate debate and discussion in this important movement in nursing and nursing education.

## A CURRICULUM FOR THE FUTURE
## OF NURSING EDUCATION

In thinking about development of a curriculum for a discipline in higher education, individuals look to the philosophy and goals of the college or university within which the program will be implemented to identify the internal factors that influence a curriculum. In addition, the external factors must be identified, such as licensing laws in the state, essential financial, human, and material resources, student population to be served, and professional and accreditation standards. Many of the curriculum principles discussed in the first part of this book are used in this section.

Recognition is given to the fact that there are several different programs leading to the first professional degree in nursing. The majority of programs follow a pattern that shows a curriculum developed in colleges and universities at the undergraduate level with a major in a field of study. Questions were raised in Chapter 7 about why nursing education has not followed other professions with education at a post-baccalaureate level. The decision of members of the House of Delegates of the American Nurses Association in 1978 noted that education for entry into the nursing profession in the future will be the baccalaureate program. Since this decision recognized the bachelor of science as the first professional degree, it will be used in this discussion of nursing as a discipline in higher education.

The older disciplines in higher education, such as biology, mathematics, philosophy, and chemistry, offer a major at the undergraduate level of education to provide a foundation for graduate study leading to a Ph.D. degree. If nurses accept the tradition of older disciplines, students would be required to pursue an undergraduate program with a major in nursing leading to a bachelor of science degree. They would enroll in a graduate program that offers a master of science in nursing and from there into a Ph.D. program in nursing. The Ph.D. would be the research degree of the discipline. If nurses believe there should be two different degrees for doctoral education, which is prevalent at this time in history, the Ph.D. is the research degree and the D.N.S. (doctor of nursing science) is the professional degree. The question arises, Is nursing an intellectual discipline? If so, isn't the Ph.D. the degree of choice, since the first professional degree would be at the undergraduate level? The purpose of the master's and doctorate in nursing would be the same as other disciplines, which is to train researchers. An example of an emerging discipline similar to nursing is education, which has offered two degrees for many years, the doctor of education (Ed.D.) and the Ph.D. in education.

The ideas suggested here are based on a philosophy that accepts the traditional approach to educational programs for a discipline. This approach is clear to academic colleagues and would clarify differences between technical education for nursing, professional education for nursing, and nursing as an academic discipline.

The discipline of nursing offers programs leading to a bachelor of science with a major in nursing, a master of science in nursing, and a doctor of philosophy in nursing. The bachelor of science program prepares individuals to become professional nurses. Continuing education provides a way to keep knowledge and skills current. The master of science in nursing offers specialization in professional nursing with emphasis on statistics, research, and computers. The doctoral program has a primary focus on research in nursing.

*The Discipline of Nursing:*
*A Hypothetical Curriculum*

The philosophy of nursing education and the conceptual framework proposed in Chapter 5 for the baccalaureate program are useful for this curriculum. The program objectives are the same with two additional objectives to be written related to the scientific method and education for health practices. The following course titles are suggested as examples of courses to be designed:

Introduction to Nursing

Historical Foundations of Nursing

Philosophical Foundations of Nursing

Conceptual Systems for Nursing

Theories for Nursing

Theories and Methods of Teaching, Learning, and Instructional Design

Diagnostic and Technical Skills in Nursing

Computers in Nursing and Health Care

Nursing of Individuals

Nursing of Groups of Individuals

Nursing in Society

Role and Functions of Professional Nurses

The following practicums would be taken concomitantly with or separate from some of the above theoretical courses:

Practicum in Nursing of Individuals

Practicum in Basic and Advanced Skills

Practicum in Nursing of Groups of Individuals

Practicum in Nursing and Health Care in Community

Practicum in Role Transition in Health-Care Systems

Following the completion of the undergraduate program, students who desire additional education would enroll in graduate programs leading to a master of science and a doctoral degree in nursing. Ideas about the kind of objectives one would be expected to achieve in graduate study are suggested below. At the completion of graduate education, graduates will:

1. Use skills of inductive and deductive reasoning and critical thinking to solve problems in nursing and health-care systems.

2. Demonstrate application of theoretical knowledge in complex and varied nursing situations.

3. Demonstrate ability to assess health states of individduals, group, and community as interrelated systems.

4. Interpret the adequacy of data in decision making in nursing.

5. Conduct research to add to nursing's body of knowledge.

6. Perform health practices conducive to a functional state of health.

7. Distinguish among rights, obligations, freedom, and responsibility in the role of a professional nurse.

8. Demonstrate ability to perform in the professional role of choice as clinician, educator, manager, or researcher.

9. Derive construct validity related to selected concepts in nursing.

10. Use of principles of learning, instructional design, and evaluation to plan, implement, and evaluate programs of health teaching for individuals and families.

At the master's level of education, individuals select an area of specialization related to age, and one nursing and health-care system. For example, health promotion may be selected as one kind of system, and adolescents would be selected as the age group. Another system may be called "coping with chronic disturbances in health state," and the age group would be adults over sixty-five years of age. Using your imagination, you can think of several nursing and health-care systems for the future that focus on individual human beings and groups rather than on disease and illness. Disease and illness are considered part of the content but would not be the major focus. The focus is human beings and their functional state of health.

At the same time that nurses are extending their knowledge and skills as clinicians, they are gaining knowledge and skills in use of research methods and designs to study problems in the individuals or groups selected as the area of specialization. At the doctoral level, the focus is on seminars to identify and study nursing problems, to develop theories, to test hypotheses generated from theories, to refine theoretical knowledge, and to study problems for immediate application to nursing situations. Instead of merely verbalizing that nurses care for the whole person or that nurses believe in holistic care, curricula are developed to provide experiences to implement these beliefs. When the focus in a program of studies is on human beings interacting with their environment, different kinds of research questions are asked than when the focus is on disease, body systems, and illness. Students also study advanced statistics, research designs, and computers, all of which provide experiences in logical thinking.

The use of the same conceptual framework for all levels of curriculum development and instruction provides structure for identifying critical variables and then organizing courses within which specific content can be identified. The overall conceptual framework used here deals with individuals, groups, and society. Added to these categories are variables of age and selected factors that influence health and nursing, such as economics, and human and material resources. The following ideas for courses for graduate education in the discipline of nursing are suggested for discussion:

Nursing and Health-Care Systems

Advanced Statistics

Computer Courses

Seminar and Practicum in Nursing of Neonates

Seminar and Practicum in Nursing of Children

Seminar and Practicum in Nursing of Adolescents

Seminar and Practicum in Nursing of Adults

Seminar and Practicum in Nursing of Older Adults (65 and older)

Measurement and Evaluation in Learning Health Practices

Research Seminar in Nursing of Neonates

Research Seminar in Nursing of Children

Research Seminar in Nursing of Adolescents

Research Seminar in Nursing of Adults

Research Seminar in Older Adults (65 and older)

Independent Study

Thesis Research

Dissertation Research

Some of the above courses would be specified for master's students, some for both master's and doctoral students, and some for doctoral students only. Variations of these groups of courses can be offered. In conceptualizing the three curricula, the focus is on individuals and groups in communities with age as a critical variable, and research as the avenue for learning and applying the scientific method to study problems relevant in nursing. A conceptually based curriculum helps learners grasp the structure of the subject rather than learn fragmented bits of information.

You may be wondering what happened to the courses in education to prepare for teaching or the courses in management to prepare for role of manager or administrator. Education, management, and administration have their own bodies of knowledge, their own theories, concepts, and questions to be solved, and they are different from those in nursing. Knowledge in these areas of study is so vast that nurses can no longer expect to take one, two, or three survey courses and become experts in teaching, management, or administration.

If nurses want to become educators, they must access that field of study to their knowledge base in nursing, because education is a profession in its own right with its body of knowledge. If nurses want to be managers or administrators, they must add knowledge from these fields of study to their background in nursing. Curricula in graduate education should be flexible so students can select courses in other fields of study to prepare them to begin to teach, manage, and be administrators. Nurses who access knowledge from fields other than nursing without the basic foundation in professional nursing will not have adequate knowledge about the profession or the discipline to teach it or to manage systems in which nursing is practiced, studied, and taught.

Within the past few years, nurses have been writing about nursing as a discipline. A review of nursing literature has shown an increase in research with some accumulation of findings to add to a body of knowledge. Conceptual systems have been constructed by individual nurses and have been evaluated in the literature. Theories have been published, and empirical testing of ideas has been initiated. The domain of nursing knowledge is receiving attention from nurses involved in this scientific movement.

Knowledge about the historical and philosophical foundations of nursing can be gained from reading the history of nursing in the United States. Two major questions have been discussed. Is nursing a profession? This question has been answered in the affirmative. A new question about nursing has been asked by nurses. Is nursing an intellectual discipline? When measured by the functions of a discipline, described by Parker and Rubin (1966), nursing is an emerging discipline in higher education. The term "emerging" is used because nursing has a short history of research as compared with other disciplines. With continued and increased efforts by researchers, nursing will be the discipline of the future.

# chapter
# *10*

# Research
# in Nursing and
# Nursing Education

The scientific aspects of a discipline go through stages in identifying the domain from which the major subject matter is identified and organized. Simply defined, a discipline is a branch of scientific knowledge. A discipline requires a group of scholars who are engaged in continuous study of problems within the domain of inquiry and who add to the body of scientific knowledge. These scholars are engaged in organizing the knowledge into the structure of the subject.

The purpose of this chapter is to highlight the importance of research in nursing and nursing education as a basis for identifying the major constructs of the nursing domain. In addition, suggestions are made about the kind of research needed in nursing and nursing education. Furthermore, ways that research can influence nursing education and nursing practice are mentioned.

## THEORY AND RESEARCH IN NURSING

Theories are the focus of science and are one of the means for discovering scientific knowledge in a discipline. The nature and structure of theories guide in the identification of the methods of inquiry in the discipline. Two elements mentioned in discussions of the structure of theories are conceptual and syntactical. Conceptual elements help identify significant questions and guide in seeking answers. Syntactical relates to the methods for studying problems in the domain of inquiry.

Shapere discussed scientific theories and their domains. He noted a series of questions should be addressed in discussing the nature of science and scientific theories. For example, what factors constitute a domain or a unified body of knowledge? Do the concepts of the domain of knowledge lead investigators to identify and study specific problems? What are the reasons for accepting solutions to scientific problems in the domain? (Suppe, 1977, p. 523).

Theories provide conceptual tools for identifying relevant questions to be studied and give direction to a research program. King's theory of goal attainment has generated hypotheses that are being tested in research in nursing practice (1981). This theory can generate hypotheses that may be tested in nursing education, such as mutual goal setting between teacher and learner. These ideas are related to a concept of mastery learning through formative and summative evaluation. Differences between norm-referenced and criterion-referenced criteria may be identified relative to goal attainment.

Theoretical formulations by nurses are being tested in different situations (Fawcett, 1984). The generation of hypotheses to test nursing theories is important in building knowledge for nursing. Programs of research must be planned to generate theoretical knowledge for nursing. Theories help define a body of knowledge for a discipline.

## DOMAIN OF A DISCIPLINE

If a discipline is a branch of scientific knowledge, then how is nursing education organized to help individuals gain that knowledge and continue to extend the body of knowledge that is used to provide an essential service? A need for research in nursing education is recognized but that need must be accompanied by the identification and agreement on the domain of inquiry in nursing. Analysis and evaluation of research of the past twenty years may be one approach for "a beginning" of organization of the body of knowledge.

If the domain of knowledge for nursing is identified as human–environment interactions that lead to a functional state of health, there is some support for this in the nursing literature and in published theoretical positions. Many concepts related to this domain have been identified. They must be tested for construct validity in nursing. If these concepts can be related to the nursing diagnosis movement, which has human–environment interactions as part of its conceptual framework, investigators would be able to conduct research to confirm a body of knowledge for nursing. Continued research will refine and extend the scientific body of knowledge. At this moment, research planned to build a body of knowledge is limited. Another question to be explored is the relationship between the concepts in the domain and the *Code for Nurses* (ANA, 1976) and the *Standards of Nursing Care* (ANA, 1973).

Several ideas for thinking about the if–then statements above are offered to stimulate discussion, debate, and critical thinking by nurses involved in the scientific movement. First, the domain of nursing appears to be gaining some consensus. Second, some common concepts are mentioned that have consistently appeared in the literature as shown in published analysis and evaluation of theoretical positions of individual nurses. Third, when the system of education for nursing is implemented that shows that the first professional degree is offered in undergraduate programs in colleges and universities, graduate education for nursing can be clarified and changed. For example, when one studies in a major field at the undergraduate level, the knowledge, skills, and values provide a basic foundation in that discipline. Graduate education builds on this foundation and leads to a master of science and a doctor of philosophy degree. Do we need the variety of titles and degrees in master's and doctoral programs in nursing that exist today?

## DOMAIN OF NURSING

Individual speeches, individual authors, and small groups of nurses have suggested that there should be one conceptual framework for nursing and it should be accepted by all as the domain of nursing. Recently, analysis of a number of conceptual frameworks has identified commonalities in the writings of individuals who have conceptualized nursing (Fawcett, 1984). Fawcett identified a framework for the analysis and evaluation of selected conceptualizations in nursing and called it the "metaparadigm for nursing" (p. 5). She explained the differences between conceptual models and theories. Her position is that a discipline may have one paradigm with a variety of conceptual models from which many theories are derived (p. 23). The four concepts in her paradigm are person, environment, health, and nursing. If nurses accept these four concepts as the artificial boundaries within which relevant questions will be asked and research conducted to answer the questions, the scientific movement in nursing will move forward with speed.

If you analyze the nursing literature of the past, you will find the same comprehensive concepts that Fawcett used to evaluate conceptual models for nursing. Many concepts developed in the literature can be subsumed as subconcepts within the four comprehensive terms identified by Fawcett. Theory development, hypotheses testing, and replication of studies are suggested as relevant areas for research in nursing. One area of research in nursing education that is limited is evaluation and measurement of student achievement of objectives. Since concepts are the building blocks for theories and conceptual frameworks, validation of concepts as substantive knowledge for nursing is an important area for research.

## CONCEPT DEVELOPMENT AND TESTING

Many concepts have been identified by individuals as relevant knowledge for nursing. For example, pain has been shown to occur in all aspects of nursing and in a variety of forms. Circadian rhythms such as body temperature, sleep–wake cycles, blood gases, and shift rotation of nurses have been studied by nurses and others since the early 1960's. Empathy has been operationally defined and studied in nursing situations by nurses (Zderad, 1968; Forsyth, 1979) for about twenty years. Concepts of movement and mobility have been studied in nursing. Concepts of interpersonal communication, space, time, self, caring, health, growth and development, stress, and many more have been identified as relevant knowledge for nursing.

Continued research may validate these concepts. A few nurses have developed some of these concepts in a review of the literature by stating the characteristics of the concept and providing a conceptual definition. In a few instances operational definitions of concepts have been given, such as for transactions (King, 1981, pp. 150–151). The literature reveals that concepts, such as stress, are developed at different levels. Individuals who have been studying stress have defined stressors and have indicated approaches for measuring stress in human beings and in nursing situations.

Several approaches for developing concepts have been published. One approach demonstrates the use of Wilson's (1963) framework; this can be found in a theory book by Chinn and Jacobs (1983). Another approach was used by King (1975, 1981) that shows a review of literature related to the concept from which the characteristics and a definition of the term were derived. The characteristics are used to observe or measure the concept in nursing situations. This process is followed by application of the knowledge gained in developing the concept in concrete nursing situations.

Another approach for developing concepts is found in a conference held in the southern region under the auspices of the Southern Region Education Board (Zderad & Belchior, 1968). At this conference Peplau presented her framework for developing concepts (Zderad and Belchoir, 1968, pp. 12–16). If one accepts the diagnostic categories in the national nursing diagnosis movement as concepts, then nurses who have consistently attended and arrived at the "defining characteristics" of each category have shown another approach for developing concepts for nursing. For further information, refinement of some of the original characteristics of the diagnostic categories was reported in the proceedings of the fifth national conference (Kim, McFarland, and McLane, 1984).

Objective testing of concepts to arrive at construct validity has been limited in published studies. Testing concepts in research provides a fertile field for nurses interested in validating relevant concepts for nursing practice and education. If the domain of inquiry is pronounced and concepts validated, then development of a curriculum for the discipline of nursing in higher education would be facilitated. Subjects would be organized around the intellectual inquiry of the discipline.

The influence of theory development, hypotheses testing,

construct validation, and replication of studies has not existed long enough in nursing and nursing education to have shown an obvious impact in the field of inquiry. When knowledge results from continued research efforts in these areas, curricula will change as the structure of knowledge for the discipline will become clear. The application of knowledge from research in nursing will help nurses provide effective care for the public.

The scientific movement in nursing during the past fifteen years has given some direction to the emergence of nursing as a discipline in higher education. Increased research will further differentiate the intellectual and professional perspectives in nursing.

## REFERENCES FOR PART III

Achinstein, P. *Concepts of Science: A Philosophical Analysis.* Baltimore: Johns Hopkins University Press, 1968.

American Nurses Association. *Report to the House of Delegates.* Committee on Long Range Goals. Mimeographed. New York: American Nurses Association, 1960.

American Nurses Association. "First Position on Education for Nursing." *American Journal of Nursing* 65 (1965), 106–11.

American Nurses Association. "Identification and Titling of Establishment of Two Categories of Nursing Practice." Resolution, House of Delegates. *American Nurse*, September 15, 1978.

American Nurses Association. *Code for Nurses.* Kansas City, Mo.: American Nurses Association, 1976.

American Nurses Association. *Standards for Nursing Practice.* Kansas City, Mo.: American Nurses Association, 1973.

American Nurses Association. *Facts About Nursing.* Kansas City, Mo.: American Nurses Association, 1982.

Bixler, G.K., and Bixler, R.W. "Professional Status of Nursing." *American Journal of Nursing* 59 (1959), 1142-47.

Bridgman, M. *Collegiate Education for Nursing.* New York: Russell Sage Foundation, 1953.

Brown, E.L. *Nursing for the Future.* New York: Russell Sage Foundation, 1948.

Bruner, J.S. *The Process of Education.* New York: Vintage Books, 1960.

Carper, B.A. "Fundamental Patterns of Knowing in Nursing." *Advances in Nursing Science* 1 (1978), 13-23.

Chance, K. "Nursing Models: A Requisite for Professional Accountability." *Advances in Nursing Science* 4 (1982), 57-65.

Chinn, P.L., ed. *Advances in Nursing Theory Development.* Rockville, Md.: Aspen Systems Corporation, 1983.

Chinn, P.L., and Jacobs, M.K. *Theory and Nursing: A Systematic Approach.* St. Louis: C.V. Mosby, 1983.

Christy, T.W. "Entry Into Practice: A Recurring Issue in Nursing History." *American Journal of Nursing* 80 (1980), 485-88.

Committee on the Grading of Nursing Schools. *Nursing Schools Today and Tomorrow.* New York: Committee, 1934.

Copp, L.A. "Nursing 2069." *Nursing Forum* 8 (1969), 82-85.

Department of the Interior, Bureau of Education. "Nurse Training Schools, 1917-1918." In *Biennial Survey of Education, 1916-1918.* Washington, D.C.: U.S. Government Printing Office, 1921, 549-646.

Department of the Interior, Office of Education. *Biennial Survey of Education, 1926-28.* Washington, D.C.: U.S. Government Printing Office, 1930, 178-189.

Department of Higher Education. *Charting the Course for Higher Education.* Washington, D.C.: National Education Association, 1951.

Donaldson, S.K., and Crowley, D.M. "The Discipline of Nursing." *Nursing Outlook* 26 (1978), 113–20.

Fawcett, J. "On Research and the Professionalization of Nursing." *Nursing Forum* 19 (1980), 310–17.

Fawcett, J. *Analysis and Evaluation of Conceptual Models of Nursing.* Philadelphia: F.A. Davis, 1984.

Fitzpatrick, J., and Whall, A. *Conceptual Models of Nursing: Analysis to Application.* Bowie, Md.: Robert J. Brady Company, 1983.

Forsyth, G.L. "Exploration of Empathy in Nurse-Client Interactions." *Advances in Nursing Science* (1979), 53–60.

Gamer, M. "The Ideology of Professionalism." *Nursing Outlook* 27 (1979), 108–11.

Ginsberg, E. *A Program for the Nursing Profession.* New York: MacMillian, 1950.

Giroux, H.A.; Penna, A.N.; and Pinar, W.F., eds. *Curriculum and Instruction.* Berkeley, Cal.: McCutchan Publishing Company, 1981.

Goldmark, J., ed. *Nursing and Nursing Education in the United States.* New York: MacMillan, 1923.

Goodrich, A. "The Nurse as Interpreter of Life." *American Journal of Nursing* 29 (1929), 427–28.

Greene, J. "Science, Nursing and Nursing Sciences: A Conceptual Analysis." *Advances in Nursing Science* (1979), 57–64.

Kim, H.S. *The Nature of Theoretical Thinking in Nursing.* Norwalk, Conn.: Appleton-Century-Crofts, 1983.

Kim, M.J.; McFarland, G.K.; and McLane, A.M., eds. *Classification of Nursing Diagnoses.* St. Louis: C.V. Mosby, 1984.

King, I.M. "A Conceptual Framework for Nursing." *Nursing Research* 17 (1968), 27–31.

King, I.M. *Toward a Theory for Nursing.* New York: John Wiley and Sons, 1971.

King, I.M. *A Theory for Nursing: Concepts, Process and Systems*. New York: John Wiley & Sons, 1981.

King, I.M. "A process for developing concepts for nursing through research." In P. Verhonick, ed. *Nursing Research*, Vol. I. Boston, Mass.: Little, Brown & Company, 1975.

King, I.M. "National Survey of Philosophies of Nursing Education." *Western Journal of Nursing Research* 6, 4 (1984). 3, 387–404.

Lambertson, E. *Education for Nursing Leadership*. Philadelphia: J.B. Lippincott, 1958.

Lancaster, W., and Lancaster, J. "Models and Model Building in Nursing." *Advances in Nursing Science* 3 (1981), 31–42.

Laudan, L. *Progress and its Problems: Toward a Theory of Scientific Growth*. Berkeley, Ca.: University of California Press, 1977.

Levi, M. "Functional Redundancy and the Process of Professionalization: The Case of Registered Nurses in the United States." *Journal of Health Politics, Policy, and Law* 5 (1980), 333–53.

Lewis, E. "The Issue that Won't Go Away." *Nursing Outlook* 27 (1979), 107.

Lewis, E. "The Professionally Uncommitted." *Nursing Outlook* 27 (1979), 323.

Longway, I.M. "Curriculum Concepts—An Historical Analysis." *Nursing Outlook* 20 (1972), 116–20.

Losee, J. *A Historical Introduction to the Philosophy of Science*. 2nd ed. Oxford: Oxford University Press, 1980.

Lynaugh, J. "The Entry into Practice Conflict: How We Got Where We Are and What Will Happen." *American Journal of Nursing* 80 (1980), 266–70.

Lysaught, J.P. *An Abstract for Action*. New York: McGraw-Hill, 1970.

McKay, R.P. "Discussion: Discipline of Nursing—Syntactical Structure Relation with Other Disciplines and the Profession of Nursing." *Communicating Nursing Research* 10 (1975), 23–30.

Montag, M.L. *The Education of Nurse Technicians*. New York: G.P. Putnam & Sons, 1951.

Montag, M.L. *Community College Education for Nurses*. New York: McGraw-Hill, 1959.

National League for Nursing Education. *Standard Curriculum for Schools of Nursing*. Baltimore, Md.: Waverly Press, 1917.

National League for Nursing Education. Committee on Education. *A Curriculum for Schools of Nursing*. New York: National League for Nursing Education, 1927.

National League for Nursing Education, Committee on Curriculum. *A Curriculum Guide for Schools of Nursing*. New York: National League for Nursing Education, 1937.

National League for Nursing Education. *Essentials of a Good School of Nursing*. New York: National League for Nursing Education, 1942.

National League for Nursing. *Minutes, Council of Baccalaureate and Higher Degree Programs*. New York: NLN. 1982.

Nutting, M. Adelaide. "Educational Status of Nursing." U.S. Bureau of Education Bulletin No. 7. Washington, D.C.: U.S. Government Printing Office, 1912.

Parker, J.Cecil, and Rubin, L.J. *Process as Content: Curriculum Design and the Application of Knowledge.* Chicago: Rand McNally, 1966.

Phenix, P. *Realms of Meaning*. New York: McGraw-Hill, 1964.

Polit, D.F., and Hungler, B.P. *Nursing Research: Principles and Methods*. 2nd ed. Philadelphia: J.B. Lippincott, 1983.

Roberts, M.M. *American Nursing: History and Interpretation*. New York: MacMillan, 1954.

Rodgers, J.A. "Toward Professional Adulthood." *Nursing Outlook* 29 (1981), 478–81.

Schwab, J. "The Concept of the Structure of a Discipline." *The Educational Record* 43 (1962), 197–205.

Shermis, S.S. "On Becoming an Intellectual Discipline." *Phi Delta Kappan* 44 (1966), 24–36.

Suppe, F., ed. *The Structure of Scientific Theories.* Urbana, Ill.: University of Illinois Press, 1977.

Taylor, E. "Of What is the Nature of Nursing?" *American Journal of Nursing* 34 (1934), 473–76.

Tinkley, M., and Beaton, J.L. "Toward a New View of Science: Implications for Nursing Research." *Advances in Nursing Science* 5, 2 (1983), 27–36.

Torres, G., and Yura, H. *Today's Conceptual Framework: Its Relationship to the Curriculum Development Process.* New York: National League for Nursing. 1974.

U.S. Commissioner of Education. *Report for the Year 1879.* Washington, D.C.: U.S. Government Printing Office, 1881.

Walker, L.O., and Avant, K.C. *Strategies for Theory Construction in Nursing.* Norwalk, Conn.: Appleton-Century-Crofts, 1983.

Watson, J. "Professional Identity Crisis—Is Nursing Finally Growing Up?" *American Journal of Nursing* 81 (1981), 1488–90.

Watson, J. "Nursing's Scientific Quest." *Nursing Outlook* 29 (1981), 413–16.

West, M., and Hawkins, C. *Nursing Schools at the Mid-Century.* New York: National Committee for the Improvement of Nursing Service, 1950.

Wilson, J. *Thinking with Concepts.* London: Cambridge University Press, 1963.

Yura, H., and Walsh, M. *The Nursing Process*. New York: Apple-
    ton-Century-Crofts, 1983.

Zderad, L.T., and Belchior, H.C. *Developing Behavioral Con-
    cepts in Nursing*. Atlanta, Ga.: Southern Regional Educa-
    tion Board, 1968.

# Index